THE
GOOD
HEALTH
FOOD
GUIDE

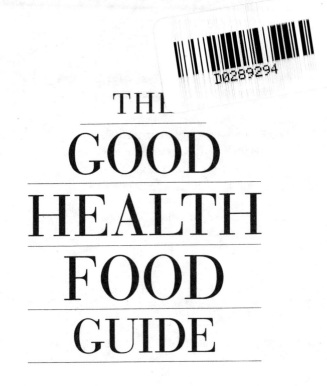

THE
GOOD
HEALTH
FOOD
GUIDE

DR ERIC TRIMMER

PIATKUS

© 1994 Dr Eric Trimmer

Published in 1994 by
Judy Piatkus (Publishers) Limited
5 Windmill Street
London W1P 1HF

The moral right of the author has been asserted

*A catalogue record for this book is available
from the British Library*

ISBN 0 7499 1138 7
ISBN 0 7499 1143 3 (pbk)

Edited by Susan Fleming
Designed by Paul Saunders

Typeset by Action Typesetting Limited, Gloucester
Printed in Great Britain by
Bookcraft Ltd, Midsomer Norton, Avon

Contents

ACKNOWLEDGEMENTS

I am indebted to my editor, Susan Fleming, for her excellent work, and also to Helen Adams, researcher, who has assiduously trudged through many a health-food shop and pharmacy that I was unable to visit and who has made most valuable analyses for me about the availability of products. To both I offer my sincere thanks.

Many pharmacists and friends from the world of nutritional science have given me the benefit of their opinions, too. Errors and omissions are, however, my responsibility.

ERIC TRIMMER
Isle of Wight

NOTE

The treatment of illness should always be supervised by a medical practitioner and you should consult your own doctor before introducing health-foods supplements into any medical regime.

INTRODUCTION

THAT there is a link between health and what we eat has been known for thousands of years. But the first really 'hard' scientific knowledge came to light only two centuries ago, when an English naval doctor demonstrated that adding citrus fruit to the ordinary daily diet could prevent scurvy. This is a disease resulting from insufficient Vitamin C, and sailors on the long voyages of the time were particularly prone to it, lacking an intake of fresh foods, especially fruits and vegetables. By adding C-rich limes and lemons to the stores on board, ships' crews were able to top up their levels of the vitamin, thus avoiding the lassitude, stiffness, bleeding gums, loose teeth and bruising that a prolonged deficiency can cause. This particular health-food supplementation led to British sailors being dubbed 'limeys', a sobriquet still applied to the British by their Australian cousins!

Thus the lemon or lime became the first acknowledged health food, a food taken to supplement levels of nutrients vital to the positive maintenance of the body and thus to good health. But it is only in the last few years that the concept of health foods has been truly pioneered. That these can make a massive contribution to positive health has been accepted enthusiastically by the public; they have been accepted much more slowly by the medical establishment. Initially the acknowledged health foods were mainly vitamin preparations: breads and flours were fortified by Vitamin D during the Second World War, and a dose of cod liver oil was the bane of many a child's day. Gradually, though, other benefits of some health foods were recognised. The original therapeutic use of cod liver oil, for instance, was as a preventative against the disease of rickets, but it is now widely recognised that it can also alleviate rheumatism and help prevent heart disease.

The list of health foods is expanding all the time. Evening primrose oil is a recent find, benefitting women particularly, and helping prevent and treat skin complaints. The valuable contribution fibre can make to the diet is a fairly recent discovery too, and 'new' remedies such as that of the herb feverfew – used in both the health-food *and* orthodox medical management of migraine – are being discovered all the time.

The Good Health Food Guide is unique in that it is the only book to examine medically and scientifically the health foods available today over the counter in health-food shops and pharmacies and, occasionally, on prescription. If you have ever walked into a specialist health-food shop, you will have found a bewildering array of products on offer. Deciding what health food might best help a particular problem, which would be the most effective variety, and how to balance that intake with other nutrients, is a huge quandary for the uninformed.

In this book, however, you will find answers. In the first part are listed the minerals, micronutrients, vitamins and other health foods which the body either needs or can find beneficial. Advice is given on deficiencies, food sources, dosage, and problems the health food can alleviate or prevent. The second part of the book approaches from the opposite angle, listing the problems or diseases that have been shown to be related to deficiency of a particular health food or which can actively benefit from an intake of individual health foods.

I have been a physician for over 40 years, and have long and intimate experience of the ills that our flesh is heir to, and what can help prevent, alleviate or cure them. I truly believe that health foods in supplement form are a new and valuable armament in the fight against disease. Although health-food manufacturers are prohibited by strict regulations from making health claims on their products, this book will tell you what the labels can't.

Why Do We Need Health Foods?

In the USA, where in many areas of preventative health care they do rather better than we do, it is estimated that 75 per cent of deaths today are due to lifestyle-related (degenerative) diseases. Of course, there's much more to *lifestyle* than eating and drinking, but whichever way you look at it, what you put into your stomach every day has a distinct tendency to turn into you. So how healthy or unhealthy you are is directly and unarguably related to the food you eat.

We would appear to be very well-off nutritionally in the West. We get enough protein to build and service our bodies, and enough carbohydrates to provide us with an abundant energy bank. But in these days of the machine, and sedentary occupations, we do not need as many calories as we once did when we led more active lives. As a result many of us can't spend enough of the energy at our disposal, and we get over-fat on 'stored' energy. We also eat too much of things that are bad for us, which allows our bodies to get out of balance. Too high an intake of animal fat, for instance, can make us prone to many fat-induced diseases (artery problems and coronary heart disease). This is one lifestyle change that has afflicted the 20th century, but health foods can help us regain a balance.

Another lifestyle change is the enormous growth of food technology in the last few decades. A really well-stocked supermarket today will carry more than ten times as many items on its shelves as did a grocery store a decade or so ago. But such apparent abundance has been purchased at a nutritional price not often realised, for the shelf product can compare unfavourably with the natural product it replaces. These negative health factors come in the form of flavour enhancers, colourings, preservatives, emulsifiers, stabilisers, and so on. Probably only about half of the food we swallow is now derived from wholesome natural foods (fresh fruit and vegetables, whole grains, lean meat, fish and milk products). The rest come from manufactured processed flour, sugar and fat products in which other considerations are rated more highly then nutritional quality.

Because we obtain over 60 per cent of our calories from purified sugars, animal fat, milled grains and alcohol, and because we process and cook (sometimes more than once) most of the food we eat, we continually hover on the edge of health needs as far as minerals and vitamins are concerned. In fact, if we ate all our food raw and unprocessed, Nature would give us four times as much vitamins and minerals every day of our lives.

The last time a really large governmental survey looked at a nation's diet in a comprehensive way was in the USA in the late 1970s. It showed that the *average* diet of the *average* American was deficient in iron, magnesium, calcium and B$_6$ vitamins, and it was assumed that many other vital nutrients might be lacking too. The same sort of deficiencies are part and parcel of our lifestyles in the whole of the civilised world today but, happily, sensible use of appropriate health foods can redirect us to a safe state of nutritional balance.

For a simple six-point plan to a healthy diet, see the Appendix.

Who Needs Health-Food Supplements?

We probably all do to a certain extent, but there are some groups of people whose needs are greater than those of others when *average* diets are consumed. The elderly, whether at home or in institutional care, hover around the borderline of malnutrition during their last decade. Often a simple nutritional supplement can bring them healthier and happier later years.

Many people have difficulty *absorbing* vital nutrients from food in the normal way, and they will probably need supplementation. Only rarely does malabsorption produce florid and dramatic symptoms. Often such poor absorbers of vital nutrients suffer from vague symptoms – a sense of feeling one degree under, with symptoms that they are ashamed to bother the doctor with. Their inherent lack of well-being only becomes obvious when they discover a health food that suddenly bucks them up. *The Good Health Food Guide* makes that process more precise and effective.

Individual absorption of and needs for nutrients are often very idiosyncratic, varying from person to person. You, your sister, your brother and your mother may well have very differing needs for various nutrients.

Experiments investigating the needs of women for Vitamin C, for instance, showed that they varied in their optimal needs between 42 and 154mg of the vitamin each day to keep them fully 'topped up'. And we now know that human needs of a whole range of nutrients change substantially with all sorts of previously ignored factors. For instance, if we eat a lot of animal-derived fat in our diet we need extra Vitamin E to keep us fit and well. Disease, stress, trauma, infection and surgery all greatly affect our nutritional requirements as well. There is a considerable body of evidence to show that in some cases vitamin and mineral supplementation far in excess of everyday needs speeds recovery if you have an operation, get involved in an accident, or suffer a nasty burn. Magnesium is now routinely given to post-operative heart patients, and Vitamin C has proved invaluable in helping the recovery of severely burned patients.

Selecting the Best Health-Food Buys

Coming to definite conclusions about particular health foods, and selecting the best, has proved to be most difficult. This does not mean, though, that the selection in *The Good Health Food Guide* has been a matter of luck. As a physician, I have included those health foods that *seem to me* to be supported by medical research to a substantial degree. I have also drawn on my own professional experience of many of the products, although a pharmacist would perhaps come to some different conclusions, as might a herbalist.

GOLD STANDARD HEALTH FOODS

In Part Two you will see that I have awarded some health foods the Gold Standard. This means they have definite benefits for a particular condition, for example evening primrose oil in the treatment of eczema (see page 227). These were easy to select. They include health foods that are supported by double blinded clinical trials published in reputable medical or scientific journals. The fact that a food or supplement does not earn this accolade does not mean that it is ineffective, however. A double blind trial means that neither the patient nor the trial assessors knows which patients are receiving placebo or product under test until the trial is terminated and codes are broken, and not all remedies and treatments can be effectively subjected to such trials.

'USEFUL' HEALTH FOODS

Some very useful health foods exist which do not or cannot conform to my Gold Standard status. There are various reasons why they have not attracted medical research, but these too have been evaluated as honestly as possible, using such supporting science as is available.

In most cases the text indicates why individual health foods are considered to be 'useful' or 'worth trying'. The rationale behind this concept of usefulness will only be appreciated if the text is taken as a whole.

RECOMMENDED BRANDS

For each health food in Part One I have, where possible, recommended specific brands. Since many products are so similar to one another this was not easy to do.

In making my choice it was reasonable to be influenced to some extent in favour of large industrial producers who *also* operated in the field of pharmaceuticals rather than the smaller, specialised health-food manufacturer. But some smaller health-food manufacturers operate systems of quality control equally as precise as the pharmacological giants, and make excellent products.

I was also looking for a product that provided *meaningful* amounts of the nutrient in question in safe, once-a-day dosage. Several medical surveys have demonstrated that patient compliance, as far as taking medicines is concerned, is at its highest when the number of times that the treatment has to be swallowed is at its lowest, so once-a-day was ideal. To ascertain whether the dosage is meaningful, look for guidance on the packets: the best products indicate the percentage of the recommended allowance that a daily-dose product allows. (*This* is the important factor, *not* the references to 'extra potency', 'super strength' etc.) I indicate what I consider to be meaningful doses, and there is information on governmental dietary values at the end of this Introduction.

When a choice exists, I usually consider tablets preferable to capsules. Tablets can be manufactured so that they provide the body with food-like properties that can be digested in a way similar to food. Enteric-coated preparations (see Glossary) in the health-food market are often unsatisfactory. Capsules are said to be 'easier to swallow' but this is a debatable and unmeasurable point. Capsules are not acceptable to vegetarians as capsule gelatin is an animal product. Also, capsules need to have an 'oily' centre unless the oil can be emulsified by means of an additive. On general principles, water-soluble health foods (eg Vitamin C and B products) are best taken in a more natural food-like tablet form, which is, incidentally, also cheaper, giving better value for money.

I believe chewable products have little to recommend them, and they can cause dental decay problems. I also view with suspicion products which lay great store in being 'natural' – all nutrients are basically natural products! Often, synthesised 'unnatural' products can be more standardised and therefore more effective. Tablet shelf-life does not seem to be a major consideration in the food-supplement world. The presence of Vitamins C and E in health foods often has a serendipitous function, inasmuch as these substances have a preservative as well as an antioxidant action and so enhance shelf-life. This often influenced my choice.

Packaging in health foods is also worth thinking about when making a choice between products. I tend to favour blister packs over bottles and canisters, particularly for those whose fingers are disabled.

Finally, although this was very difficult, I attempted to opt for 'value for money' preparations wherever possible. Coupled with this was a factor that only dawned on me towards the end of my 'good buy' task – the 'readability' of the pack information. My optician claims that provided I wear the right glasses my vision is perfect. If I had to 'screw-up' my eyes to read the product information on the pack, this influenced my choice too!

EXCESSIVE CONSUMPTION

Concern over this often influenced my choice of product. One of the advantages of a packaging that expresses dosage in relation to the percentage of the recommended daily intake is a built-in protection against overdosage. Unfortunately changes in Department of Health policy are making this safeguard less easy to apply.

Overdosage is only a real worry in a handful of nutrients, and high on this list is Vitamin D, and it is wise not to exceed its Dietary Reference Values (see the box on page 142). Vitamins A and D have potentially dangerous properties if they are consistently taken to excess, mainly because the body is capable of storing these substances to a greater or lesser extent. Some health-food enthusiasts take several products concurrently with differing health aims in view. In such cases it is wise to do a total A and D count to prevent overdosage. Because beta-carotene is a precursor (see Glossary) of Vitamin A in the body, and is also non-toxic, it may prove safer than Vitamin A as a health food.

Overdosage with the water-soluble Vitamins B and C is unlikely to produce health problems except in two instances. Doses of pyridoxine (Vitamin B_6) in excess of 50mg per day have been associated with temporary impaired function of sensory nerves – although, for this to occur, usually large doses (2 – 7 grams per day) have been involved. High doses of the water-soluble vitamins are, generally speaking, a waste of time and money, for the body quickly excretes mega doses.

Large regular doses of Vitamin C have sometimes been followed by scurvy-like symptoms on cessation of mega therapy – a practice that has in itself little to recommend it in any case.

One point I feel is worth remembering is that some people's bowels are quite easily upset by the nutrient or the excipients (that 'glue' the nutrients together) when they opt for a course of dietary supplement. Usually this minor inconvenience can be avoided by gradually building up the dosage, perhaps by taking the tablet every other day or by making experimental alterations to the time of taking the supplement relative to eating food. Products available in smallish (trial) packs often influenced my Good Buy choice.

How to Use This Book

First of all, read the section in Part Two (A – Z of Illnesses and Complaints) that interests you. Each entry concludes with examples of useful health-food Good Buys, and, where appropriate, Gold Standard products (see page 11). Then read the appropriate sections in Part One (A – Z of Health-Food Supplements). These will fill in the detail and help you to choose wisely from what is available in the health-food shop or pharmacy. I truly believe and hope that this will save you time and money, improve your health, and promote a greater sense of well-being.

Measuring Nutrients

Different units can be used to measure nutrients and this can cause confusion, for example when comparing labels on products.

You may see nutrients expressed in one of three ways:

- **milligrams** (abbreviation mg)
  There are 1,000 milligrams in one gram

- **micrograms** (abbreviation µg. Sometimes shown on products as mcg)
  There are 1,000,000 micrograms in one gram
  There are 1,000 micrograms in one milligram

- **international units** (abbreviation iu)
  These were introduced as an attempt to express vitamins in terms of biological activity, and are now being phased out. Here are the equivalent values in micrograms or milligrams for those nutrients that you may still see expressed in ius:

  1 iu Vitamin A = 0.3 micrograms (of retinol – see Glossary)
  1 iu Beta-carotene = 0.1 micrograms (of retinol)
  1 iu Vitamin C = 50 micrograms
  1 iu Vitamin D = 0.025 micrograms
  1 iu Vitamin E = 1.0 milligrams (of δλ alpha tocopherol acetate – see Glossary)
  1 iu Thiamin hydrochloride = 3 micrograms

15

THE NEW DIETARY REFERENCE VALUES

Most health foods still express their essential contents in the terms of Recommended Daily Allowances, or RDAs. In the future this well-known term will be less widely used in the UK, and nutrients will be appraised in a variety of forms, mainly, it would seem, to get away from the word *Recommended*. The new terms are:

• **Estimated Average Requirement (EAR)**   This is a new Department of Health estimate of the *average* requirement or need for food energy of a nutrient. Many people, it is admitted, will need *more* than the average and many people will need *less* to keep them in optimum health.

• **Reference Nutrient Intake (RNI)**   This is an amount of a nutrient that is enough for almost every individual, even someone whose needs for the nutrient are high. This level of intake is, therefore, considerably higher than most people *need*. If individuals are consuming the RNI of a nutrient, it is argued, they are unlikely to be deficient in that nutrient. You could look at it as a 'safety first' intake of a nutrient.

• **Lower Reference Nutrient Intake (LRNI)**   This is defined as the amount of a nutrient that is enough for only a small number of people with *low* needs. Most people will need more than the LRNI if they are to keep fit. If individuals are habitually eating *less* than the LRNI, they will almost certainly be deficient, given time. You might well look upon it as a low-warning level of nutrient intake.

• **Safe Intake**   This is a term normally used to indicate the intake of nutrients for which there is not enough information to estimate exact requirements. A safe intake is one which is judged to be adequate for almost everyone's needs but not so large as to cause undesirable effects.

• **Dietary Reference Values (DRVs)**   A general term used to cover all the figures produced by the Department of Health Panel – LRNI, EAR, RNI, and safe intake.

All DRVs, the Department of Health points out, are intended to apply to *healthy people*; they do not make any allowance for the different energy and nutrient needs imposed by fickle eating, disease, disability, old age or institutionalisation. By using the word 'reference', the Department hopes that we will not interpret any of the sets of intake figures as being *recommended* or *desirable* intakes. Somehow or other, it is hoped that we, the consumers of foods and nutrients, will use the most *appropriate* set of figures for any *given situation;* and use them as a general point of reference rather than as definitive values to be etched on to the nutritional consciousness of the nation. Is this a helpful attitude? Will it foster a more sensible attitude towards eating and the consumption of dietary supplements? Time alone will tell.

The relationship between various reference values is expressed graphically below.

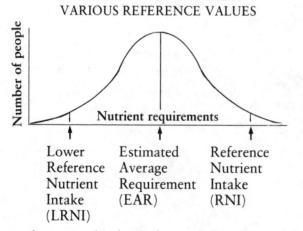

RELATIONSHIP BETWEEN
VARIOUS REFERENCE VALUES

Number of people

Nutrient requirements

Lower	Estimated	Reference
Reference	Average	Nutrient
Nutrient	Requirement	Intake
Intake	(EAR)	(RNI)
(LRNI)		

The author puts this book forward as a research-based, personal statement and guide for those who wish to know more about health foods. If a reader has health worries about disease, then a doctor should be consulted.

Part One

A–Z OF
HEALTH-FOOD
SUPPLEMENTS

CALCIUM

THERE is more calcium in the body than any other mineral, and 99 per cent of it is found in your bones and teeth, where it not only forms the mass of these organs but acts to some extent as a store or reservoir. The body regulates its blood calcium content by means of a special hormone system which keeps about 10g of calcium liquid in the blood and tissues, leaving over a hundred times as much on deposit in the bones and teeth.

Signs and Symptoms of Deficiency

Calcium deficiency sometimes declares itself as symptoms in the form of otherwise inexplicable muscular aches and pains, an irregularity of the heart's action, or attacks of palpitation. More frequently the prime sign is osteoporosis (brittle bones) and periodontal disease (gum recession and tooth loosening). Weight-reducing diets which are low in milk, bread and cheese, the most common sources of dietary calcium, can bring about deficiency problems. Pregnant and lactating women, and women who are involved in hormone replacement therapy, probably benefit most by taking some extra calcium.

Do You Need Supplementation?

If you are trying to reduce your fat intake, as medical and nutritional experts are advising the population of the Western world to do, then you may need to think about your diet. Those who are following advice to eat with their cardiovascular health, their gall bladders, or even their shape in mind, will often logically exclude the fat of milk and cheese - the major sources of calcium – from their diet as far as possible. But it is possible to minimise the low-fat = low-calcium equation by replacing ordinary milk with skimmed or low-fat milk and low-fat cheese. The fat level is reduced, but the calcium level remains the same.

Calcium is absorbed in the small intestine, and this absorption requires Vitamin D. A low-calcium diet can thus be compensated for by the presence of Vitamin D. Anything that hurries the food along through the small bowel (fibre, roughage) hampers calcium absorption, but Vitamin D mitigates this.

Phytates, which occur in wheat, form insoluble salts with calcium and therefore inhibit its absorption if the wheat foodstuff is of the unleavened variety, e.g. *chapattis*. (For foodstuffs to be absorbed they have to be soluble.)

— FOOD SOURCES —

Milk; cheese (Cheddar and cottage); yoghurt; ice cream; white bread (in which case calcium is *added* during flour manufacture); pulses; cabbage and certain other leafy green vegetables; canned sardines; white fish.

Hard water can supply a fair proportion of adult needs.

INSOMNIA AND CALCIUM

A milky drink is often the solution to sleeplessness, and milk contains significant amounts of calcium. Supplementation could just help a chronic insomnia problem.

OSTEOPOROSIS AND CALCIUM

Osteoporosis is a disease of bone, which occurs with ageing. Bones in the body become less well nourished, lose mass and become brittle and liable to fracture. The tendency is particularly common in women who have gone through the menopause, when hormonal balances in the body are altered.

Calcium is a major constituent of bone, and therefore a diet rich in calcium, plus a supplement, is indicated.

PERIODONTAL DISEASE AND CALCIUM

A loss of bone mass in the jaw, which holds the teeth, can lead to widening and infection of the gum margin, and to subsequent teeth loosening. Calcium foods and supplements, as above, can help.

Dosage, Contraindications and Side Effects

The average dietary intake of calcium in the USA is 450–550 mg (UK figures are roughly similar), and yet the RNI (Reference Nutrient Intake) for calcium is 700mg per day. As RNIs are designed to meet the needs of only 95 per cent of the population, it would certainly seem sensible for everyone to increase their calcium intake, perhaps up to 1,000–1,500mg a day, in the interests of maintaining a positive balance of calcium all the time. This would combat one cause of osteoporosis, for instance. It is important to make sure that a really low calcium intake is always avoided. If intake falls below 250mg a day only 70 per cent of calcium is absorbed, and it is easier to *lose* bone strength than to *gain* it.

However, increased intake of calcium leads to progressively reduced rates of absorption. There is little convincing evidence that any benefit would accrue from intakes higher than 2000mg daily, which are sometimes recommended for the prevention or treatment of osteoporosis. But because high intakes of calcium are not generally associated with any detrimental effects, it is prudent for those at particularly high risk of osteoporosis to take diets which are rich in calcium.

Dietary supplementation with elemental calcium poses a potential problem due to the possible encouragement of kidney stone production, particularly in those with a predisposition to or history of stone formation. Similarly, if magnesium supplementation is being pursued with a view to reducing the likelihood of suffering from kidney stone disease, taking a combined calcium/magnesium supplement would not be indicated.

GUIDANCE ON INTAKES

DRVs (Dietary Reference Values) for Calcium, mg per day

	LRNI		EAR		RNI	
Age	Males	Females	Males	Females	Males	Females
15–18 yr	450	480	750	625	1000	800
19+ yr	400	400	525	525	700	700

Additional amounts to be added to pre-pregnancy DRVs
Lactating women + 550

Note: Menopausal women should probably take a supplement, but the Department of Health has not endorsed this at present.

GOOD BUYS

Most calcium supplements are relatively low in calcium content. Good buys contain more than rival products.

Osteocare (VITABIOTICS)

Contains 300mg of calcium combined with magnesium, zinc and Vitamin D to aid absorption and utilisation in the body.

Calcia (ENGLISH GRAINS HEALTHCARE)

Contains 750mg of calcium carbonate and various vitamins and minerals to aid absorbtion.

NHS PRESCRIPTION PRODUCTS

There are several calcium preparations prescribed by doctors under the NHS, including:

CaCit (NORWICH EATON)

Caldichew (SHIRE)

Calcidrink (SHIRE)

Calcium Sandoz (SANDOZ)

They are all good buys containing relatively high calcium doses.

CALCIUM AND MAGNESIUM COMBINED

Some nutritionalists stress the inter–relationship of magnesium and calcium. Dr Mildred Seelig, a world authority on magnesium, believes that when osteoporosis does not respond to calcium and Vitamin D, then supplements of magnesium are necessary. Several companies supply a combination of these minerals – Healthcrafts, Natural Flow, Quest, etc.

Magnezie (LIFEPLAN)
This is a balanced combination of 150mg of calcium and magnesium together with a complete range of minerals plus B vitamins and Vitamins C, D and E. It is a one-a-day supplement and is available from most health stores or by mail order from Lifeplan.

Dolomite (CANTASSIUM)
Dolomite contains calcium and magnesium in natural mineral combination of calcium 28 per cent and magnesium 13 per cent.

Balanced Ratio Cal-Mag (QUEST)
Contains 100mg of calcium and magnesium together with Vitamin D.

See also: **Magnesium; Vitamin D; Insomnia; Menopausal Problems; Osteoporosis; Periodontal Disease.**

COBALT

THIS micronutrient, or trace element, is essential for human nutrition for it forms part of the Vitamin B_{12} molecule, a deficiency of which occurs in the disease of pernicious anaemia. Deficiencies can arise in undernourished communities, especially in pregnant women and in Vegans. Cobalt as such is not used therapeutically, Vitamin B_{12} being more practical.

Cobalt contained in health foods appears to have no really useful function.

See also: **Glossary.**

COD LIVER OIL

EVENING primrose oil can justly claim to have been a breakthrough in health foods, for it focused attention on the fact that there might well be unsuspected nutritional qualities associated with certain fats – the essential fatty acids (see Glossary) – other than their calorific content as high-grade energy body fuel. But cod liver oil can claim comfortably to be the oldest and most-tried health food, and still is one of the most effective products available at the health-food counter.

To some extent, this 'tried and tested' image has been somewhat of a disadvantage, for it is often thought of as old-fashioned, and has been ignored as a result. The taste has always been a disadvantage too, but this has recently improved (by instant harvesting of the liver of the cod in a factory ship at sea, which minimises the chemical changes in the oil which bring on the fishy flavour).

Do You Need Supplementation?

The oil first gained its reputation years ago, as a very effective dietary supplement containing Vitamin D as a preventative against the disease of rickets, and was 'suffered' by generations of children in the early 20th century. The oil was the richest known source of Vitamin D at that time.

When in the 1960s, the British government of the day decided to phase out cod liver oil as a rickets-preventing welfare food (in favour of a cheaper source in the form of synthetic Vitamin D), one of the largest producers (British Cod Liver Oils, or BCLO) sought other sales opportunities for their product. For ye6ars, management and scientists at BCLO had been privately convinced that there was more to cod liver oil than a possibly unpalatable source of Vitamin D. One reason for this conviction was an enormous and spontaneous correspondence that the company received which claimed that cod liver oil improved health in all sorts of other ways.

Medical and scientific minds had great difficulty in taking this on board, and it was not until the substances called prostaglandins (see Glossary) were discovered that they could start to understand how something as old-fashioned and mundane as cod liver oil could possibly have any therapeutic effect on diseases.

Cod liver oil is very rich in an essential fatty acid with a particularly awkward name, *eicosapentanoeic acid* (EPA for short). This substance is very much involved in the prostaglandin function that centres around blood 'stickiness' and clotting, and the internal chemistry of joints. So if you have blood vessel disease, arthritis or rheumatism, or if you are at risk from rickets, cod liver oil can be very beneficial. There is also a suggestion that gall bladder problems can be alleviated by EPA, particularly by cod liver oil, supplementation.

— FOOD SOURCES —

See Marine Oils, page 83.

ARTHRITIS, RHEUMATISM AND COD LIVER OIL

The most frequent of BCLO's spontaneous testimonials were to improvements occurring in a variety of rheumatic complaints. An army of sufferers constantly bombarded their offices in England's fishing city of Hull, claiming firmly that 'cod liver oil helps my aches and pains'. Eventually the prostaglandin connection between cod liver oil-derived prostaglandins and rheumatism/arthritis pathology was unravelled.

THE BLOOD-CLOTTING DISEASES AND COD LIVER OIL

The blood-clotting diseases – which encompass coronary thrombosis, stroke illness and various other vein and artery thrombosis syndromes – remain the major killers of our age. The ultimate reasons why this is so remain ill-understood, despite an enormous amount of research time, money and energy being expended.

Research indicates that the cause of blood-clotting diseases is multifactorial. Some of the major factors seem to be totally unrelated to diet – for instance smoking, blood pressure, genetic or inherited tendencies, stress, excessive alcohol intake and poor exercise habits. But it is becoming increasingly acknowledged that diet is also closely linked to all thrombosis diseases and is, in all likelihood, related to our prostaglandin intake.

As is so often the case in medicine, chance observations made by scientifically-oriented individuals are frequently followed by scientific progress. It was the research done by the British nutritional scientist. Hugh Sinclair that opened the medical establishment's eyes to the life-saving virtues of marine oils in general, and to cod liver oil in particular. He firmly believed that an increase of essential fatty acids in the diet and a reduction in *non*-essential fatty acids, is vital to prevent blood-clotting diseases.

Only very gradually is modern medical management proceeding along these lines. In the mean time cod liver oil stands as an extremely valuable health food.

Dosage, Contraindications and Side Effects

The dosage, as for marine oils (see page 83), depends on how much fish you regularly eat. It is virtually impossible to overdose on cod liver oil as it contains relatively little Vitamin D. This can be a potential hazard with halibut liver oil (see page 84).

Cod liver oils and other marine oils should not be taken by anyone known to have a bleeding disorder – haemophilia or recurrent nosebleeds – and should not be taken in conjunction with anti-coagulant therapy. It is inadvisable to take marine oils when undergoing dental treatment involving extractions.

The only reported adverse reactions are occasional nausea and belching.

GOOD BUYS

Seven Seas Range
Cod liver oil capsules are available in various-sized packs. A one-a-day super or high-strength capsule is available; ordinarily you have to take several capsules to obtain a 5ml dose.

Pure liquid cod liver oil is available for people who do not mind the taste of the oil or for those who dislike swallowing capsules. The bottle has an easy-open cap for those suffering from arthritis. Various-sized bottles are available.

A cherry flavouring in one liquid oil combats the fishy taste. Orange syrup cod liver oil is a blend for growing children or anyone who would like the fishy taste of the oil masked by a sweeter flavour. The orange syrup form also contains Vitamins A, D, E and C and B_6 at safe recommended levels.

Other Products
High-grade cod liver oil, in capsule and liquid form, is also available from several other reputable manufacturers including Boots and Healthcrafts. MAXEPA (Novex) is a type of 'super' cod liver oil, and is prescribable under the NHS.

See also: **Glossary; Marine Oils; Plant Oils** and **Artery Problems; Arthritis and Rheumatism; Cardiac Problems; Gall Bladder Problems; Rickets.**

COENZYME Q10

CHEMICALLY, Coenzyme Q10 or CoQ10 is a quinone, a member of a brightly-coloured cyclic organic group of biologically active compounds much involved with intracellular energy exchange. The highest concentrations of CoQ10 occur in the organs of the body in which energy exchanges are maximal, e.g. the heart and the liver. It used to be expensively extracted from offal (heart and liver), but comparatively recently, pharmacological synthesis has made it cheap enough to reach the health-food market.

Several hundred scientific papers have been published in recent years on various aspects of CoQ10's pharmacology, many of which have focused on its capacity to restore impaired immune functions, improve cardiac function, and favourably influence the progression of chronic neurological syndromes.

It has become known as the 'energy enzyme', and as such, can be taken for quite a number of problems.

ALZHEIMER'S DISEASE (AD) AND COENZYME Q10

CoQ10 has been used fairly extensively in treating many AD patients, with some minor success, so it is definitely worth trying.

PERIODONTAL DISEASE AND COENZYME Q10

In trials, supplementation with CoQ10 seemed to restore gingival health, and a number of studies have reported favourably on its use.

TIREDNESS AND FATIGUE AND COENZYME Q10

Because of its 'energy' boosting abilities, CoQ10 is gaining quite a reputation as an anti-tiredness remedy.

GOOD BUYS

Coenzyme Q10 (HEALTHILIFE, WASSEN)

COPPER

THIS interesting micronutrient, or trace element, is most likely to be found in the health food shop in *macro* form as a copper bangle from which copper in micro amounts is absorbed via the skin. Copper is, indeed, essential to our diet, and we need perhaps 1.2mg per day. It is necessary for the formation of oxygen-carrying haemoglobin, although the element does not appear in the actual haemoglobin molecule.

Signs and Symptoms of Deficiency

Adult humans rarely suffer a deficiency, unless living exclusively on processed foodstuffs. Babies whose mixed feeding is delayed beyond six months can suffer a deficiency, resulting in diarrhoea followed by anaemia, as cows' milk is a poor source of copper.

— FOOD SOURCES —

Liver; shellfish; green vegetables; nuts; wheat; pulses; unrefined grains; dried fruit; tap water in some soft-water areas.

ARTHRITIS, RHEUMATISM AND COPPER

Interest in copper as a micronutrient in humans centres on the enzyme super-oxidase dismutase – an enzyme containing both copper and zinc. A Danish study which involved injections of the enzyme was enthusiastically received by the arthritis sufferers involved and was found to be both safe and effective. Two other US trials have shown super-oxidase dismutase to be as 'effective as gold injections but without the side effects'.

Most rheumatologists are unconvinced that percutaneous absorption of copper helps in the management of rheumatism, although so many wearers of copper bangles are convinced of their efficacy. It has been suggested that copper from copper bracelets augments the action of antirheumatic drugs like aspirin, phenylbutazone and indomethacin.

Dosage and Side Effects

Large doses (250–500mg per day) are toxic. A safe intake is suggested to be 1.2mg per day.

There is some evidence that side effects from excessive intake include extreme fatigue, irritability, multiple muscle pains and headaches. A few multiple-mineral health foods contain copper, but overdosage of copper is more likely to follow drinking water from the hot-tap in soft-water areas in which copper plumbing is joined together with lead solder materials.

GOOD BUYS

A good buy containing a suitable daily supplement of copper is marketed as Genesis (Wassen). It also contains comprehensive supplementation of most vitamins, minerals and micro-nutrients.

EVENING PRIMROSE OIL

APART from keen horticulturalists, very few people knew much about the evening primrose until comparatively recently. Plant historians first found it growing around dockland areas, its seeds having arrived accidentally in cargoes from North America. 'Evening primrose' is a good descriptive name, for the plants look a bit like large primroses, with yellow flowers that open in the evening and last for about a day.

Just before the end of the First World War, it was found that the plant's seed was rich in an oil quite different from the fatty substances found in many other seeds. This was gamma linolenic acid, or GLA for short, the 'superstar' among essential fatty acids (EFAs, see Glossary). But more than 40 years elapsed before British scientists showed much interest in the oil's health potential.

Do You Need Supplementation?

The essential fatty acids content, particularly the GLA, of evening primrose oil is one of the *essential* key factors in our body for the efficient production and distribution of certain hormone-like chemical messengers, the prostaglandins (see Glossary).

— FOOD SOURCES —

Apart from 'specialised' seed sources, GLA is found in corn (wheat, maize etc.), soya beans, olives and fresh leaf vegetables. It is easily destroyed by 'ageing' and oxidation.

As to how much you might need, it is extremely difficult to be dogmatic on this point. To some extent, this depends on how much GLA you obtain from your normal diet – and this is very variable (see Food Sources). Variable too are the so-called GLA-blocking factors (pages 326–7). Any one of these may mean you need extra GLA in your diet on a daily basis to make sure that the vital prostaglandins involved in maintaining optimum health are around all the time, for unfortunately your body cannot store them. Most authorities believe that a good, safe, dietary supplement to maintain optimum health is around 480mg GLA daily.

WOMEN AND EVENING PRIMROSE OIL

Women have been realising for some time that by taking a daily dose of evening primrose oil they can often benefit their general well-being. It can alleviate the less pleasant symptoms of pre-menstrual syndrome, or prevent recurrent breast pain at period times. The oil also has a distinctly beneficial effect on the general condition of the skin and nails, and so GLA itself has also gained something of a cosmetic reputation. This difficult-to-define 'hidden' health-bonus factor is something that seems to differentiate certain highly reputable health foods from other less effective products.

ECZEMA AND EVENING PRIMROSE OIL

Eczemas often involve allergy. Patients who suffer from skin allergies (for instance, to washing-up liquids, solvents, plants or flowers – even, on occasion, to sunshine) are all suffering fundamentally from a problem of enzyme blockage in their biological pipeline at the stage at which linolenic acid is converted in the body into GLA. This leaves them relatively deficient in the substances that the body further builds into the prostaglandins involved in maintaining skin health. Evening primrose oil, as capsules or skin oil, can be very helpful.

An interesting focus on GLA as a skin-health provider comes from the study of babies who suffer from eczema. Many such babies are, in fact, really demonstrating an allergy to cows' milk and again GLA intake is involved. Human milk is pretty rich in GLA, but cows' milk and most formula feeds (which are made from cows' milk) are very low in GLA. Modern treatment of baby eczema is proceeding logically along the lines of giving GLA-rich evening primrose oil as a dietary supplement, or by actually rubbing it into the baby's skin.

But favourable results in adult trials are even more significant: the skin improved dramatically, and skin itching decreased.

Evening primrose oil is Gold Standard therapy for all allergic type eczemas.

FIBROCYSTIC BREAST DISEASE AND EVENING PRIMROSE OIL

Trials have demonstrated that the pain of this disease can be significantly reduced by supplements of evening primrose oil.

HYPERKINESIS AND EVENING PRIMROSE OIL

An interesting hypothesis has been put forward that links hyperkinesis (hyperactivity in children) with essential fatty acid (EFA) intake, for it has been suggested that many foods which seem to be implicated in hyperkinesis symptomatology are weak inhibitors of the necessary conversion of EFAs into prostaglandins within the body (see Glossary). This may go some way towards explaining the male preponderance of hyperkinesis, for males are known to have higher EFA requirements than females.

Hyperkinetic children often suffer from other well-known EFA deficiency problems (eczema, asthma and allergies), and this has led to EFA-based studies being mounted. Good preliminary results have been recorded in hyperactive children when given 1 – 1.5g of evening primrose oil twice daily.

MULTIPLE SCLEROSIS (MS) AND EVENING PRIMROSE OIL

There is an increasing body of evidence to suggest that EFA-rich polyunsaturated oils can be beneficial to MS sufferers, reducing attacks and prolonging remissions. Evening primrose is one such oil.

Dosages, Contraindications and Side Effects

Please see Plant Oils, page 85, for advice on dosage. If GLA products are being taken for gynaecological symptoms, gynaecological cancer should be excluded by means of an examination.

Schizophrenics should not take GLA products except under medical supervision, and neither should epileptics or those taking drugs who are predisposed to fits (your doctor or pharmacist will advise).

No major adverse reactions have been reported, although some takers complain of nausea, indigestion and headaches.

GOOD BUYS

Evening Primrose Oil Company (EPOC) Range

There is a variety of capsules, the size describing the amount of oil contained. All have Vitamin E as well. (The rationale for this is to provide an antioxidant bonus, and to act as a stabiliser, thus increasing the shelf-life of the product.)

There is also a 15ml bottle of EPOC liquid, a pure evening primrose oil with Vitamin E. This is supplied with a special dropper, and is useful for treating children with eczema.

Efamol Range (BRITANNIA HEALTH)

The Efamol evening primrose crop is grown in the UK as well as certain places in Europe where climatic conditions favour a high GLA content; a back-up crop is grown in New Zealand. The basis of the range includes capsules and a pure oil. The 250mg capsules are helpful for children or those with swallowing difficulties. The pure oil is deal for external application to the skin, but can also be taken internally (10 drops are equal to one 500mg capsule). This product is suitable for both vegetarians and Vegans, and has been approved by the Vegetarian Society.

Efamol Plus contains 250mg of evening primrose oil as well as 200mg of safflower oil and 50mg of linseed oil. This combination provides additional polyunsaturated fatty acids for further dietary supplementation.

Efamol Marine combines the benefits of 430mg of evening primrose oil with 107mg of marine fish oils. (These have a rather different 'therapeutic window' from that of plant products, see Marine Oils, page 82.)

The *Efamol Pre-Menstrual Pack* contains ten days' supply of Efamol 500mg capsules plus Efavite tablets. The tablets contain co-factors such as Vitamin B_6 which help ensure the full utilisation of the essential fatty acids in Efamol.

Healthilife Range
This is a high-quality range which consists of pure evening primrose oil capsules. There is also a roll-on applicator for external use, plus a cream, which are good buys in eczema or dermatitis situations.

Boots Range
Boots market a useful range of evening primrose oil products.

See also: **Glossary; Marine Oils; Plant Oils; Allergy; Artery Problems; Arthritis and Rheumatism; Eczema; Multiple Sclerosis; Pre-Menstrual Syndrome.**

FIBRE

DIETARY fibre is best defined as the structural residue of plant foodstuffs that is undigested by the time it reaches the large intestine. Chemically there is not just one substance called fibre, for plant structure is a very variable entity; the many 'fibres' are composed of carbon, hydrogen and oxygen and are therefore chemically carbohydrates – cellulose, pectin, lignin and hemicellulose, for example.

But because fibre is non-digestible, as far as we humans are concerned (lacking the fibre-digesting enzyme of ruminant animals), it provides the necessary bulk to the stool to maintain an easy and efficient bowel transit. Fibre also absorbs a lot of water which keeps the stool soft and easy to pass (1 gram of fibre can bind up to 15 grams of water).

Despite the early enthusiasms of such medical philanthropists as Sylvester Graham in the USA (after whom Graham Crackers – a wheat flour product broadly similar to Digestive biscuits – were named), Dr T.R. Allinson in the UK (who was the inspiration of the famous flour company), and a young American doctor called John Harvey Kellogg, it was not until the 1920s that the medical professions of the world started to look at food with particular reference to its fibre content, and to relate disease to lack of fibre in the diet.

In most industrialised nations there has been a prevailing trend towards the increasing consumption of low-fibre foods (food processing decreases fibre content). A whole gamut of eating-pattern changes has brought this about, and fibre depletion in our diet has occurred together with a corresponding increase in constipation and the associated conditions of diverticulosis, colon cancer, and probably irritable bowel syndrome, too.

Fibre Today

The most recent news about fibre comes from a Department of Health publication, *Dietary Reference Values*, a guide prepared by Jenny Salmon for the Department of Health, London, 1991. It suggests that we should abandon the term dietary fibre for a new term, NSP (non-starch polysaccharides). This is in order to define more accurately the type of chemical compounds that we call fibre, and to standardise a method of analysing them so as to reach a sensible conclusion about how much of these NSPs we should include in a healthy diet. The panel responsible for the Department of Health's publication came to some very sensible and straightforward conclusions that are well worthy of consideration here.

1. A daily intake of NSPs in excess of the average consumption today would be desirable.
2. NSPs help to lower blood cholesterol.

3. NSP intakes of less than 12g per day are associated with bowel disorders such as cancer and gallstones.

4. Some NSP components, however – especially those in wheat bran – contain the substance phytate which may bind with minerals such as calcium, iron, magnesium, zinc and copper, and so make them, theoretically at least, unavailable to the body. Thus care and dietary supplementation need to be taken, especially by the elderly and those whose diets are only marginally adequate in such minerals.

5. There appears to be no virtue in exceeding an NSP intake of 32g per day.

Do You Need Supplementation?

To some extent this depends on what sort of foods you enjoy eating, whether you have your own teeth or not (some fibre-rich foods can be difficult to chew!), and what sort of metabolism you have. Certain fibre-rich foods give some people an uncomfortable type of intestinal gas indigestion (although iron can occasionally help, see page 72). Many people also experience food-allergy problems, and find that certain foods just upset them. (To a large extent it is advisable to come to terms with the fact that if, for instance, green peppers or kidney beans upset you, it is best *not* to try to eat them.)

— FOODS HIGHEST IN FIBRE —

Natural bran and bran cereals; baked and dried beans, and peas, pulses and grains; wholemeal bread, crisp-breads and brown rice; dried fruit (especially prunes); green leafy vegetables (eat raw or cook very lightly); baked potatoes (eat the skin); fresh fruit (especially bananas); nuts.

Sometimes how much we can eat of a fibre-rich food is dictated by the number of calories that it is wise for us to consume each day, and in cases like this, fibre-rich low-calorie health foods or 100 per cent bran is clearly the answer.

Happily there is one fairly good indication that we are or are not eating enough fibre. The large, fibre-rich stool that comes with an adequate fibre intake will float rather than sink in the lavatory pan, and so the right dosage of the right type of fibre is really just a case of simple trial and error.

BOWEL CANCER AND FIBRE

Cancer very rarely occurs in the small bowel, but cancer in the large bowel is the second commonest cancer in the West. High incidence of colon cancer is a comparatively recent occurrence in our society – the disease was rare in the 1920s, for instance. Bowel cancer tends to be more rare in rural communities than it is in urban areas and in cities. These simple and undisputed facts have led to speculation about possible links between diet and large bowel cancer. The main difference between diet in truly rural communities and urban ones is that the former diet contains more fibre and less fat.

Although there is no promise implied that if you eat a high-fibre diet (and one that is low in fat) you will escape colon cancer risks, there seems to be sound reasoning for increasing fibre intake on the grounds of cancer prevention.

CONSTIPATION AND FIBRE

The useful role that fibre can play in bowel motility-related conditions, has produced a therapeutic revolution in the orthodox medical management of constipation. Many of the 'old' stimulant laxatives have been virtually abandoned by the medical profession in favour of nutrient or health-food laxatives, although a few old-style laxatives are still good sellers in pharmacies and health-food outlets.

The most natural way of curing constipation is to increase the amount of fibre-rich foodstuffs in the daily diet. However, the extra fibre in the food taken should not be an overwhelming source of calories. Bread, for instance, is suspect, not because it is all that rich in calories, but because of the highly calorific things like butter, margarine and jams that so often accompany it. Fruit and vegetable fibre is preferable. Bran, which is virtually non-calorific, heads the list of useful fibre-rich foods and is often the key to health-food constipation management.

CROHN'S DISEASE AND FIBRE

Crohn's is an inflammatory bowel disease, and a fibre-rich diet has been shown to be helpful. The water-absorbing and bulking abilities of bran help to prevent irritation of the bowel, and to make the stools firmer.

DIABETES AND FIBRE

Many studies have indicated that high-fibre diets improve what is referred to as glucose tolerance – in other words, it edges the diabetic's reaction to glucose in the diet in the direction of normalcy. Diabetics who increase their fibre intake *may* be able to decrease their insulin or tablet medication under medical supervision. It has been noted that diabetes is rare in 'primitive' societies in which the population eats large amounts of fibre and small quantities of simple sugars as part of the diet.

GALL BLADDER PROBLEMS AND FIBRE

Gallstones can cause medical problems, and fibre could help. An experimental controlled study group of thirteen patients with proven gallstones ate a diet containing variable amounts of fibre daily to see what effect this would have on a test called the bile-saturation index (a test of predictability for gall-bladder disease). This was found to be higher in the low-fibre periods of diet. In other words, fibre has a protective effect on gallstone formation.

Another study of healthy individuals, who simply added 50g (2oz) of wheat bran per day to the overall diet for four weeks, showed a significant decrease in their bile cholesterol and their bile-saturation index – both indicators of gallstone risk.

(Vegetarianism has been proven to be associated with a lower incidence, 50 per cent, of gallstones.)

HYPERTENSION AND FIBRE

Hypertension – or high blood pressure – can cause minor distress or contribute to major accidents such as stroke, coronary problem or heart failure. Although the reason is not properly understood, fibre – whether as fruit or vegetable, or as bran – has been shown to reduce blood pressure. A study of health food shoppers (see page 245) who were asked to eat an extra 100g (4oz) of fibre per week, revealed small, but significant, falls in pressure.

IRRITABLE BOWEL SYNDROME (IBS) AND FIBRE

Most studies evaluating the effect of bran in the management of IBS were small, experimental and controlled, and are somewhat equivocal in their results. One placebo-controlled study showed a significant reduction in symptoms on bran therapy at 12 weeks but this tailed off at 16 weeks. The fact that IBS symptoms come and go makes evaluation difficult.

VARICOSE PROBLEMS AND FIBRE

Both haemorrhoids or piles and leg varicose veins are commonly thought to be caused by pressure being transmitted to the veins when defacating, especially when constipated. A diet rich in fibre could prevent varicocities forming, and help relieve haemorrhoid discomfort if it is present.

Dosage and Contraindications

See Fibre Today, page 37.

GOOD BUYS

Fibre products are more likely to find their way into the diet from the grocer or supermarket than via the health food counter.

A best-buy evaluation is difficult in view of the lack of product standardisation, but simple low-calorie products are to be particularly recommended. Linusit Gold is good.

A good working principle is if the product tastes sweet, then check for its sugar content. If this is substantial, seek a product with a lower sugar content.

Linusit Gold (FINKS)
Linusit consists of organically grown linseeds, and is rich in both soluble and insoluble fibre, essential fatty acids and minerals. The seeds are split open before being packaged and retain maximum effectiveness with the minimum of processing. Because of its gentle but highly effective action, it is suitable for women who experience constipation during pregnancy. Linusit can be sprinkled onto yoghurt, cereals, soup and stews, or used in a variety of ways.

Natural Country Bran (JORDANS)
This is natural wheat bran, and it contains the outer layers of the wheat grain, minerals and enzymes. Each 100g contains 49g of fibre, as well as 100mg of calcium and 600mg of thiamin.

Oat Bran (JORDANS)
This contains both oat bran and oat germ. An analysis of the main nutrients per 100g shows 15g of dietary fibre, as well as 14.5mg of iron, 3.8mg of zinc, 3.7mg of thiamin, and 3.3mg of Vitamin E.

High Fibre Biscuits (GRANNY ANN)
These are excellent for a savoury snack, especially as each biscuit contains 5g of fibre. They come in two varieties but contain raw sugar or date syrup. Granny Ann also make High Oat Bran Biscuits which include fibre.

GF Dietary, Rite-Diet (NUTRITIA DIETARY PRODUCTS/ JUVELA)

This includes a range of fibre products for those with food sensitivities, including a sensitivity to wheat or gluten. Rite-Diet High Fibre Bread is gluten-free, and a product called Beta Fibre can be used to make up a variety of pastries or cakes.

Apple Fibre Chewable Complex (BLACKMORE'S)

This product is low in calories. Each tablet contains 400mg of wheat bran, 400mg of psyllium husk powder, 200mg of powdered apple and 50mg of apple cider vinegar powder. It is free of all artificial sweeteners, yeast, milk derivatives, preservatives, artificial colours and flavours. The only group of people who would not be able to take it are those sensitive to wheat products.

NHS PRESCRIPTION PRODUCTS

There are several of these available, and doctors have a wide choice of prescription. Two bran-based products are **Trifyba** (Sterling Winthrop) and **Fybranta** (Norgine).

See also: **Cancer; Constipation; Crohn's Disease; Diabetes; Gall Bladder Problems; Hypertension; Irritable Bowel Syndrome; Varicose Veins, Ulcers and Haemorrhoids.**

FLUORIDE

FLUORIDE is an interesting micronutrient, or trace element, in that it is not essential for humans or the lower animals, but is a substance that by its presence prevents, or at least gives some protection against, dental caries.

Perfect teeth can be formed in the presence of very low concentrations of fluoride, but about 1 part per million in the water supply definitely delays the development of dental caries. Water supply authorities will advise customers over the telephone as to the presence or absence of fluoride in their supply. In non-fluoride areas dental protection can be obtained by taking fluoride tablets, painting the teeth with a fluoride solution by the dentist, or using fluoride toothpaste.

Excessive fluoride is thought to be deposited in bone, but there seem to be no health hazards involved in this. It is possible that there may, in the future, be other health bonuses. Fluorides bind to aluminium in the Alzheimer victim's brain and if a definite link between aluminium intake and Alzheimer's Disease is identified, then clearly dietary supplementation with fluoride will become very interesting.

Dosage and Contraindications

Around 5mg per day is thought to be a safe intake. Tea drinking often provides sufficient intake as tea is rich in fluoride (as is fish skin). But if a 'chain' tea drinker makes tea with fluoridated water, a mottling of the teeth – or fluorosis – can result. This is when fluoride, instead of enhancing the tooth enamel, actually damages it.

GOOD BUYS

Fluor-a-Day (DENTAL HEALTH)

Fluoriguard (COLGATE-PALMOLIVE)

GARLIC

ALTHOUGH garlic has been used as medicine since ancient times, it is a comparative newcomer to the world of health foods. Said to have originated in Siberia, the plant has been grown widely in the Latin countries bordering on the Mediterranean for many centuries. It was not used in cooking in the UK until after the Second World War, when wider travel in Europe started to change conventional British gastronomic tastes. Even now there are many who will not countenance its inclusion in dishes, let alone think of it as medicinal. But an advertisment in the *Morning Post* (a national newspaper in 1922) had a curiously modern ring to it, for it recommended 30 drops of an alcoholic extract of garlic as a remedy for 'arterial' tension (presumably high blood pressure).

CARDIAC HEALTH AND GARLIC

An interest in the geographical facts related to the risk of having a heart attack has awakened an interest in garlic as a medicinal substance. It has been shown that the worst places to live in the UK if you want to avoid a heart attack are Central Scotland or West Yorkshire, areas that are rumoured not to rate garlic very highly in the kitchen. It could be said that in those areas they smoke and drink too much, or they lead lives that are too stressful, and that the lack of garlic has nothing whatsoever to do with it. However, it is possible to find in western Europe areas that match the 'black spots' of Scotland or West Yorkshire rather well with reference to general social environment and habits but which enjoy better cardiovascular health.

The French, for instance, have a relatively low incidence of the ischaemic heart disease (where blood flow is restricted) that produces so much coronary thrombosis in those who live on our side of the Channel. The smoking and alcohol patterns of the two nations are really very similar and, of course, both nations are heavily industrialised and show similar stress factors. They also have a very similar fat consumption. Is it possible therefore that the relatively high culinary garlic consumption in western Europe plays a part in protecting its residents from heart attacks? This problem was recently examined in depth in the *British Journal of Clinical Practice* under the editorship of the consultant physician to the West Middlesex University Hospital, and gave considerable support to the concept of garlic as a cardiovascular prophylactic.

HYPERTENSION AND GARLIC

Every doctor agrees that one of the multifactorial causes that increases the risks of developing artery disease is a raised blood pressure. Thus many health educational bodies are devoted to the concept of *lowering* high blood pressure. In Europe one such body is the German Hypertension League, which has promoted changes in behaviour and healthier eating, and changes involving relaxation schemes and exercise schedules. If this was not effective, specific therapy was advised but using low-risk plant preparations.

Trials conducted using a commercial garlic extract of *Allium sativum* (Kwai) have recently been carried out to test this hypothesis. An excellently designed trial was organised by the Professional Association of German Practitioners. It involved 47 groups of non-hospitalised patients suffering from mild hypertension, and was placebo-controlled, randomised, double blind and conducted over a period of 12 weeks. During the trial, blood pressure and blood lipids (chemical indicators of coronary disease proneness) were monitored. Statistically significant differences in blood pressure were found in favour of garlic takers over those taking the placebo.

Another double blind trial was carried out at the University of Hanover. This involved 40 patients who had raised blood cholesterol levels (another indicator of coronary disease proneness) as well as higher than healthy blood pressure. It demonstrated without doubt that powdered garlic in a 900mg daily dose significantly lowered blood cholesterol and other blood-related risks as well as the actual blood pressure when compared to a placebo control group.

Do You Need Supplementation?

Yes, if high blood pressure problems and risks of coronary disease are to be minimized.

Odourless garlic preparations are readily available on the shelves of most health food shops. For those who prefer the real stuff, include it in a variety of Mediterranean-style dishes. One clove of garlic per day is a reasonable intake.

Side Effects

Although garlic appears to be completely non-toxic, some people find it upsets their gastro-intestinal tract. Sometimes food allergy occurs. Often the sufferer can be gradually desensitised to garlic either as food or supplement by starting with minimal doses and gradually increasing the dose. Sometimes enteric-coated garlic helps as well.

GOOD BUYS

As there have been no comparative trials with reference to garlic and garlic products, it is impossible to be dogmatic about a relatively good buy. There is nothing to suggest that manufactured products are better than the natural product from the prophylactic point of view, but for those who cannot tolerate the side effects of fresh garlic, such products offer certain advantages.

Neither are there any RDAs or other 'official' dosage recommendations. It should be pointed out that the German trial mentioned above used a relatively high daily dose (900mg powdered garlic).

Kwai – Highly Concentrated Garlic Tablets (LICHTWER PHARMA)

These garlic tablets are produced in Germany, by a process of drying and gently slicing the cloves which leaves the finished product as near to the real thing as possible and retains its important therapeutic properties. The highest grade of

47

organically grown Chinese garlic cloves are used. The tablets are completely odourless, and free from artificial colour, preservatives, flavourings, starch, salt or gluten. The product is relatively expensive.

Kyolic Range (QUEST)
The Kyolic range is produced from organically grown garlic. The products are totally odourless, rich in nutrients from whole garlic, and cold-aged without heat. (Cold-ageing is thought to preserve the essential oils.) Natural garlic is sun- or heat-ripened.

Kyolic 404 is a daily 'preventative' garlic supplement. The tablets are formulated in a base of oat bran and lecithin, without the use of any animal products, and so are suitable for Vegans.

Kyolic 100 is a relatively expensive product. It is suitable for vegetarians, and contains 300mg of garlic.

Kyolic 102 is suitable for Vegans and contains 350mg of garlic.

Healthilife Range
Mega Garlic Pearls, each capsule of which provides 0.66mg of odourless garlic powder.

One-a-Day Odourless Garlic Pearls, each capsule of which provides 2mg of odourless garlic powder.

Cardiomax (HÖFELS)
Recently popular, a low-odour one-a-day supplement of concentrated garlic oil plus a little peppermint oil to aid digestion. Each capsule contains the equivalent of six cloves of garlic. It may prove useful for those who cannot tolerate garlic.

One-a-Day (delayed diffusion) Garlic Tablets (WASSEN)
A useful once-a-day preparation.

Odourless One-a-Day Garlic Oil (BOOTS)
A reasonably-priced product.

See also: **Artery Problems**; **Cardiac Problems**; **Hypertension**.

GINSENG

GINSENG shares a somewhat mysterious reputation with a handful of other health foods. Generally speaking, the majority of the medical profession opine that because they cannot understand *how* ginseng works therapeutically they are inclined to conclude that it does *not* work. They also say that the various claims made for ginseng in the world of dietary medicine are very definitely not proven.

Of course, it might be *just* possible that a medicinal plant which has held a place of high esteem among takers for over 4,000 years is totally useless, but this would seem rather unlikely. Rather more likely is that we in the West have a deep inbuilt suspicion of everything Oriental. For even sceptics find the medical history of ginseng difficult to ignore. Its reputation as a medicine began in Asia where it is widely used in the management of anaemia, diabetes, insomnia and neurosis. In China it is taken as a tonic and revered as a source of general health, strength and happiness. It is considered especially useful for the aged, and as an aphrodisiac.

The generic name for the ginseng plant is *Panax*, which is derived from the Greek words meaning 'panacea' or 'cure-all'. There are at least three types of ginseng, all botanically members of the plant family *Aralia*. Originally the 'best' ginseng was thought to come from Manchuria, but today it is cultivated widely throughout the world, and it is doubtful if any one form is very much better than another.

All ginseng plants are rather unimpressive perennial shrubs, and the active principle is found in its carrot-like roots. These are washed and sun-dried and are then eaten either *in toto* (in doses of between 0.5–3g daily), or ground up to make powders and capsules.

Does Ginseng Work?

Analysis of the constituents of plant remedies is extremely complicated. A boost to this sort of intricate chemical detective work came in the 1960s when a process known as 'thin layer gas chromatography' was developed, which disclosed many of the inner secrets of plants' chemistry. It is now generally accepted that the active principles of ginseng's complex chemistry are substances known as saponins, at least 13 of which have been isolated. Many of these have hormone-like effects on the body.

Scientific evidence of ginseng's therapeutic efficacy is not over-strong, but there is some that is difficult to ignore. High on a short list of factors suggesting an actual pharmacological action is the existence of a condition known as the 'ginseng abuse syndrome'. In other words, 'abusers' suffer a ginseng 'high'.

Some years ago the late Sir Derek Dunlop, a noted physician, said in defence of a remedy being newly introduced into clinical practice, 'Show me a drug without side effects and I'll show you a drug that does not work.' The existence of side effects occurring in ginseng takers would in itself seem to indicate that there *are* physiological changes in takers that are very definitely the result of pharmacological action.

TENSION, STRESS AND GINSENG

Ginseng was investigated at the Institute of Biologically Active Substances in Vladivostok, in what used to be the USSR. It was found to increase the ability of laboratory animals to survive previously unacceptable levels of different types of stress. The Russians coined a name to describe this property of ginseng, and referred to it as an *adaptogen*, because it seemed to help the already extant coping skills to *adapt* to greater stresses. It enhanced natural physical capabilities, and increased resistance to trauma.

These results were considered interesting enough medically for the Soviets to mount some further experiments. In one, *physical* stress was tested: 100 soldiers taking part in a cross-country marathon run were divided into two groups, one half of which took ginseng, the other a dummy tablet. The ginseng takers had better times for their runs to the extent of 12 per cent. Another experiment explored an alleged *mental* property of ginseng, to promote alertness and foster concentration. They used proof-reading as a controlled test, and once more ginseng seemed helpful and the ginseng takers spotted typesetting errors 51 per cent more efficiently than did readers taking dummy tablets.

But perhaps the most extensive ginseng experiments have involved military personnel, and as a result both Chinese and Vietnamese troops were issued with prophylactic ginseng before going into military action. Russian cosmonauts also take ginseng prior to and during space travel as an antidote to stress, which otherwise tends to impede their physical performance.

One explanation of ginseng's reputation as an aphrodisiac is that many instances of poor sexual function are related to sexual performance *anxiety*. Ginseng's 'adaptogen' property dilutes sexual anxiety and therefore allows sexual functioning to blossom naturally. Many ginseng takers find the remedy more palatable than sex counselling and sex therapy.

TIREDNESS, FATIGUE AND GINSENG

Part of ginseng's general tonic effect is to combat tiredness, and it is particularly valued for this in the Orient.

MENOPAUSAL PROBLEMS AND GINSENG

Hormone replacement therapy (HRT), when well-managed medically and carefully prescribed, is an enormously effective form of treatment for a proportion of menopausal women. Not all find HRT acceptable, however, and many such women turn to ginseng as a natural health food remedy.

There seem to be two good reasons for this. Ginseng's *adaptogen* quality helps to enhance the victim's coping skills, allowing her to come to terms more easily with the physical aspects of her new way of life. Another factor is the apparent pharmacological relationship between the chemical constituents of ginseng and certain human hormones, or at least that ginseng seems to act upon the body in a hormone-like way.

As the compounds used for HRT are sex hormones, many of them plant-derived, this could explain why ginseng is used by so many women during menopause. That fact alone should surely earn it a special place here.

Dosage and Side Effects

In common with many other 'natural' health-food remedies, ginseng does not appear in any reputable Western National Pharmacopoeia (except in Russia and Switzerland). To gain such an entry, large-scale planned research, followed by publication of reports of trials that satisfy research pharmacologists in the USA and in Europe generally, would be necessary. But because ginseng is not a patentable substance, expensive research by pharmaceutical companies is unlikely because of a lack of any patent profit motive. Thus ginseng lacks an authoritative pharmacology.

However, ginseng should not be taken in excess of 2g of dried root daily, for there are well-substantiated side effects.

In women ginseng takers, breast tenderness and swelling of the breasts is reported often enough to be notable. A sudden rise in blood pressure occurs in some ginseng takers, too, even after a short course of treatment, and so regular takers would be wise to arrange for their blood pressure to be monitored. A feeling of stimulation – a ginseng 'high' – is often reported, and quite rarely this proceeds to nervousness, sleeplessness and diarrhoea if excessive quantities are taken. One pharmacologist felt that the sense of well-being generated by ginseng might cause elderly or convalescent patients to 'over-do it' during what should be a quiet recovery process, and that suitable restrictive warnings should be given.

Contraindications

Some pharmacologists have suggested that ginseng contains an oestrogen, in which case, ginseng theoretically should share similar contraindications with the oral contraceptives (thrombotic diseases, certain cancers). Hard scientific evidence on this score is not forthcoming, however.

GOOD BUYS

It is difficult to make the best value judgement with reference to products as equivocal as the various ginsengs, but the following have developed good reputations. The Korean producers of ginseng are attempting to standardise their product, and eventually it may be possible to be more scientific with reference to *Good Buys*.

When deciding upon which is a *Good Buy* for you, the relative prices of reasonably long-term therapy (two to three months) should be taken into consideration.

Red Kooga (ENGLISH GRAINS HEALTHCARE)
Red Kooga is a popular product which is readily available and of good quality Korean ginseng. The range consists of tablets, capsules, elixir and tea. Ginseng tea comes wrapped in individual packets, each containing 3g of instant tea powder.

Power Ginseng GX2500 (POWER HEALTH)
This has been on the market for more than a decade, and is popular with athletes as an aid to stamina and endurance. The type of ginseng used is Panax CA Meyer – Korean Ginseng Root, claimed to be one of the best in the world.

Healthcrafts Range
Healthcrafts produce a wide range of products and make use of both Korean and Siberian ginsengs. Korean ginseng is recommended for maintaining physical performance, while Siberian is thought to help with mental performance and stability. It is difficult to accept the rationale of this concept.

The range consists of a blend of both ginsengs, various strengths of both Korean and Siberian ginseng, plus a supplement in two strengths containing Siberian ginseng as well as Vitamins E and B_6. The latter is targeted for the menopause. All products in this range are free of artificial colours, flavours and preservatives, yeast, gluten, lactose, salt and sugar.

Other Products
Boots and Seven Seas also produce good ginseng products.

Windsor Healthcare produce Pharmaton, which contains ginseng. This illustrates poly-pharmacy in an intense form. It is an expensive attempt to weld together many important and effective health foods. It remains a popular health food that has stood the test of time, but is unlikely to be enthusiastically endorsed by doctors generally.

HERBALIST PRODUCTS

OVER the centuries, herbal plants have provided us with a living foundation upon which modern medicines have been built. The 17th-century Jesuits learned how the Indians in Peru treated malaria successfully with a herbal remedy made from the bark of a tree: cinchona bark and its extracted alkaloid, quinine, are still used today. Foxgloves used in herbal medicine to treat heart failure eventually gave us the synthetically-produced digitalis medicines of today. About 2,000 years ago in India, Brahmin medicine used the plant *Rauwolfia*, the essence of which was developed into certain psychotrophic drugs and blood-pressure treatments. Modern orthodox medicine has now replaced them with other pharmaceuticals that are safer and more effective. Willow bark (*Salix alba*) was known to the ancients to reduce fever, and was originally a herbal remedy until its active principle was synthesised in 1860 and subsequently developed as the anti-rheumatic 'aspirin'. Opium from the seed capsules of the poppy, *Papaver somniferum*, has been used as a painkiller from the earliest times.

So, herbalism has been around for a long time. The *Great Herbal* of China appeared in about 3000 BC, and 'modern' herbalism was established in Britain by Act of Parliament during the reign of Henry VIII. The basic thought that seems to lie behind the concept of herbalism – that Nature has a cure for everything if only you seek it out – has changed little as the years have passed. In 1960 Dr D.C. Jarvis, a GP from Vermont in the USA, re-focused many people's minds on herbal remedies in his book, *Folk Medicine*, when he reminded readers that animals 'know unerringly which herbs will cure what ills', and advised his patients to heal themselves with a daily dose of honey and apple cider vinegar.

You may well be tempted to seek out your own herbal products, and Jill Nice's guide, *Herbal Remedies* (see References) contains many remedies to be found in the health food departments. And there are, of course, many plants which are valuable in medicine, some already given a place in this book – garlic and ginseng, for example. It is important, however, not to believe that just because a remedy is a herbal product that it will automatically be free of any of the potentially worrying side effects and toxic reactions that bedevil orthodox medicine from time to time. In fact, poison centres operating on a worldwide basis are slowly collecting and collating dangerous side effects associated with the ingestion of many herbal remedies in fashion today.

Throughout this book I am at pains not to take a disdainful attitude towards 'cures that work' and are thus popular with those that have faith in them, just because it is not understood how they *could* work from the scientific and pharmacological points of view.

The following is a short list of herbally-based bestsellers liable to be found on the shelves in your local health-food shop or community pharmacy, with brief comments upon the rationale that has led to their formulation.

Antifect (POTTERS)

One of the constituents of this hayfever remedy is elder, a plant that was so prized that a 1644 book stated quite simply that every part of the tree was medicinal, and that it covered 'every ailment from toothache to the plague'. More modern herbalists stress its purgative action, and the 'dehydrating' action of a purgative may well be one way in which it combats the symptoms of hayfever.

Antifect also contains garlic, which is often used by herbalists to treat asthma, a hayfever-related disease.

Biostrath Elixir (POTTERS)

This is an arthritis remedy whose herbal pedigree includes prickly ash, a very popular herbal remedy for chronic rheumatism containing xanthoxylin, thought of highly enough to be included in the US Pharmacopoeia (but apparently unresearched). Other ingredients are elder flowers and yarrow, which do not seem to have any antirheumatic property. It also contains poke root, another American 'green' remedy for chronic rheumatism that has mild narcotic properties, burdock root, an antirheumatic that dates from the Middle Ages, and other constituents that do not appear to have any known specific antirheumatic action. It is difficult to understand how it sustains its antirheumatic reputation in the market place.

Cardiomax (HÖFELS)

A garlic oil, soya bean and peppermint herbal combination formulated to promote cardiac health. (*See also:* **Garlic.**)

Feverfew (LIFEPLAN, HEALTHWISE)

The first mention of feverfew (*Tanacetum parthenium*) appeared in Gerard's classic *Herbal* of 1636, but as a herbal medicine it has been used since the Middle Ages to treat fevers. Recently feverfew has been subjected to double blind, placebo-controlled trials and has acquitted itself handsomely in the treatment of migraine. In one trial published in the *Lancet*, organised by the University of Nottingham, treatment was taken in capsule form (each capsule contained two dried feverfew leaves) as a single daily dose. Those taking feverfew experienced a reduction in the number of migraines and severity of attacks, including vomiting. There were few side effects (the commonest of which was mouth ulcers), and there appeared to be no drug interactions or contraindications. A similar trial carried out at the City of London Migraine Clinic and reported in the *British Medical Journal* disclosed similar results and a 70 per cent success rate. This makes feverfew a Gold Standard herbal remedy.

Feverfew seems to work by altering prostaglandin action in the brain. It has to be taken as a preventative – not as a treatment for the migraine attack. Many herbalists, and indeed migraine clinics, advocate the taking of fresh leaves – in a sandwich, say. The herb is a pretty lime green, and grows easily in temperate gardens.

Floradix Formula (SALUS)
The main ingredients of this are yeast, kelp, wheatgerm, rosehips and iron. It could make a fair contribution to many of the body's vitamin and mineral needs, mostly from herbal sources.

Höfels Garlic and Parsley (HÖFELS)
For the action of garlic, see Garlic. Parsley roots and seed contain *apiol*, another herbal substance that suffers from under-investigation. It has a diuretic action which may well reinforce the action of garlic.

Lanes Kalms (LANES)
Contains some of the ingredients of Lanes Quiet Life (see below), together with gentian. Gentian is another medical herb of great antiquity, being in wide use before the Christian era. In pre-tranquilliser days doctors often combined it with phenobarbitone as a general sedative, particularly for menopausal women. Modern herbalists claim the active principles in gentian root to be 'excellent tonics' that are useful in the management of 'hysteria and female weakness'. No convincing pharmacological evidence exists to support this, but on herbalists' terms of reference both of Lanes' tranquillising products would seem to be of value.

Lecigran (LANES)
This is a soya bean lecithin product which is put forward as a 'true, natural good concentrate which lowers blood cholesterol and increases brain activity'. It is difficult to see how lecithin can claim any special kudos as a herbal medicine, for it is difficult to construct a diet that is *deficient* in lecithin – eggs are a rich source, for instance. Lecithin is a health food with little to support a theory that there is anything very special about it.

Natra Calm (ENGLISH GRAINS HEALTHCARE)

An alcoholic extract of *Passiflora incarnata*, a herbalist tranquilliser which has as its active principle a substance called passiflora, thought to be similar to morphine but not addictive.

Ortizan Laxative (ORTIS)

This is a herbal laxative, the main active ingredient of which is senna. Senna is a herbal laxative of great antiquity (from at least the 9th century AD), obtained from leaflets of *Cassia acutifolia* or *C. augustifolia*. Senna produces a single-thorough bowel evacuation within six hours, and is the gentlest of the stimulant laxatives.

Disadvantages are habituation, and its 'griping' action.

Peppermint (OBOKJAERS)

Peppermint oil has recently found favour with gastroenterologists in the medical treatment of the irritable bowel syndrome (IBS). Peppermint was used by the ancient Greeks and Romans. The active principle is peppermint oil, a constituent of menthol, a substance which causes a sensation of cold in the mouth. Medicinally, peppermint oil has for long been classified as a calmative, something that 'settles' the stomach and intestine generally. Menthol is also useful as a local anaesthetic in painful sore throats, and is inhaled with steam for catarrh. Peppermint tablets are sucked by dyspeptics.

Quiet Life (LANES)

In an attempt to put together an effective herbal tranquilliser, Lanes have combined many herbs that appear to have a psychotrophic or calming action. These include hops, which are mildly sedative, motherwort, which has a reputation for 'allaying nervous irritability and inducing quiet and passivity of the nervous system', and *Passiflora incarnata*, a herbal antihypertensive. It also includes valerian, a herbal tranquilliser *par excellence* that has been prescribed by herbalists since Culpeper's day, and which, until comparatively recently, was widely prescribed by orthodox doctors. Valerian is a herb which cries out for a more scientific evaluation.

Rio Amazon Guarana Elixir (RIO AMAZON)

This has a reputation of being a quick pick-you-up type of tonic. Guarana is a South American shrub that has enjoyed a tonic reputation for over 200 years. The seeds are processed like coffee and made into a tonic. Brazilian miners drink it routinely, and it is said to be the secret ingredient of cola-type drinks. Herbalists claim it to be an aphrodisiac, a nerve tonic and a 'narcotic stimulant', although the latter claim would seem to be pharmacologically impossible. What is possible is that guaranine, which is similar to caffeine, has a therapeutic effect which should be scientifically evaluated. The elixir also contains antioxidant Vitamin E (see Vitamin E and Glossary).

Vegetable Cough Remover (POTTERS)

A stimulant to the liquification of mucus containing many herbs with an expectorant action. The most likely effective ingredient is ipecacuanha, which is called 'the roadside sick-making plant' in Brazil where its use was discovered in the 1680s. (Many expectorants 'work' due to reflex gastric irritation.) Another constituent is lobelia, named after the 17th-century botanist, de Lobel, and which has an expectorant and anti-wheezing action. Pleurisy root, *Asclepias tuberosa*, is another herbal expectorant in this product, which is also said to help the pain of pleurisy and encourage sweating.

See also: **Constipation; Hayfever; Irritable Bowel Syndrome; Migraine; Tension and Stress.**

HOMOEOPATHIC PRODUCTS

THERE are understandable reasons for the presence and popularity of homoeopathic remedies now appearing at health-food counters, both in pharmacies and in health-food shops. But to understand why homoeopathic medicines are so very different from other forms of medication you have to appreciate how very different are the two *principles* of practice.

Orthodox medicine is based on the concept of disease taking place inside the body as a result of some noxious process. Sometimes the aetiological factor is understood well, sometimes hardly at all. Treatment is designed to restore the health *status quo* by a variety of logical means (drugs, surgery, physiotherapy, transfusion, radiotherapy and so on), by neutralising the basic disease process.

Homoeopathic medicine puts forward an entirely different concept. From the beginning of medical time, doctors have noted that certain drugs will produce certain unexpected signs and symptoms when they are administered. Modern medicine calls these 'side effects'. The father of homoeopathy, Dr Samuel Hahnemann, a Leipzig physician in the early 19th century, called such effects a *similimum*, and postulated that every disease has a *similimum* in the world of Nature that, if properly administered, will cure. There is nothing scientifically logical in this *credo*. Having launched the theory, Hahnemann set about 'proving' it by experimenting with thousands of substances, and slowly but surely a homoeopathic pharmacopoeia evolved.

From the very beginning homoeopathy's pharmacopoeia was very different from any other method of therapy in all sorts of ways. To start with it employed a very different concept of dosage. In orthodox medicine, a dose is calculated in most cases around the amount of the drug given related to the weight of the patient. Often, too, deference is given to the *degree* of effect that is looked for. In other words, if you have a *bad* pain or a *heavy* infection, you need a heavier dose of your painkiller or antibiotic than would otherwise be necessary.

In homoeopathy things are quite different. For example, if you were suffering from scarlet fever in Hahnemann's day, he would have prescribed aconite because he had 'proved' that aconite had, as a side effect, a tendency to make you go red in the face, sweat and look as though you were running a temperature. Thus aconite became the homoeopathic *similimum* for scarlet fever. But Dr Hahnemann was no fool. He did not want to make his scarlet fever patient worse due to aconite side effects, so he reduced the aconite dose considerably. Strangely he found that the more he *diluted* the *similimum* the more 'powerful' was its effect. This led to the whole concept of homoeopathic prescribing – not measured in terms of quantity of the substance prescribed but by its *degree* of dilution. This produced the paradox of *potentiation* of homoeopathy in action depending upon the *minimisation* of the dose prescribed.

At this point conventional medicine tends to 'blow the whistle' in the 'homoeopathic game'. But I have only partially stated the case for homoeopathy. Part of the process is the initial consultation that takes place between you and your homoeopath, which is quite a lengthy process. It involves a probing homoeopathic history-taking and, if your homoeo-path is also a doctor, a conventional medical history and examination, too. Space prohibits any further detail here, but at the conclusion of this initial consultation another fundamental homoeopathic canon is defined – the concept of there being a *constitutional homoeopathic remedy* for you that will always help if you are ill. In other words you 'are', in homoeopathic jargon, a *pulsatilla*, a *belladonna* or a *bryonia*, for instance. By now, of course, orthodox medicine has not only blown the whistle, it has also left the field.

To the convinced homoeopath, however, the concept of a constitutional remedy is highly attractive. It provides you with a constant 'therapeutic friend' that will help at any time and for any ill. This is then reinforced if necessary with the skilful selection of a more specific remedy, a short selection of which follows, based on the practice of one of Britain's foremost homoeopathists, the late Dr Margery Blackie, physician to HM The Queen.

I was lucky enough to meet and be trained practically in

homoeopathy by Dr Blackie, who was at the time keen to introduce orthodox physicians to the art. At the time I had decided to relinquish a 25-year commitment to full-time general practice and become a part-time partner in a new practice. This gave me two new opportunities – to become editorial director of a firm of medical publishers and have the time to explore a new practice of medicine as a medical homoeopathist while still practising as a general practitioner in the NHS. To start with I was extremely sceptical of my new medical expertise. What was more depressing, I soon found, was the type of patient coming to see me, best described by the phrase 'given up by doctors'. Three of these early patients stick in my mind – a child with a depressive illness, a man with Parkinsonism and a little girl with terrible eczema. To my utter amazement, my no doubt inept homoeopathic involvement with these cases was followed by a totally unexpected degree of success. Suddenly I understood how Dr Hahnemann must have felt and why his concept of medicine is alive and well at the health-food counter today!

Margery Blackie's Homoeopathic Favourites

Acacia
For stabbing pains in the back and for ankle problems.

Acidum phosphoricum
For children's diarrhoea.

Aconite
For the sort of cold that you 'catch' by getting chilled. Also for muscular strains and nasty cuts.

Allium cepa
For the acute, watering eyes, streaming type of cold.

Argentum nitricum
For vertigo, fear of falling. Also before exams, public speaking, stage fright.

Arnica
A very popular remedy to prevent and treat muscular stiffness. Also used to stop bruising after injury and speed post-traumatic sports injury recovery.

Arsenicum
For the 'run down', and for fear and depression in the elderly.

Baryta carbonica
For enlarged tonsils.

Bella-donna
For colds complicated by sore throats.

Bryronia
For rheumatism aggravated by cold, dry weather.

Calcarea carbonica
For children who sweat profusely. Also for school phobia and slow learners.

Capsicum
For ear problems in children (glue ear).

Carbo vegetabilis
For wind and gastric distension.

Causticum
For piles, anal fissure, or for loss of voice.

Chamomilla
For the difficult baby with teething troubles, the infant who seems constantly at odds with the world, demands mother's attention, and 'irritable' adults.

Cinchona
To elevate mood.

Cocculus
For travel sickness.

Colchicum autumnale
For gouty, rheumatic complaints.

Gelsemium
To counter tension before examinations, stage fright, tendency to rely on alcohol to combat nervousness, rumbling dyspepsia.

Graphites
For infantile eczema.

Hepar sulphuris
For infantile eczema.

Hyoscyamus
For senile dementia, depression and 'awkwardness'.

Hypericum
For post-traumatic neurosis.

Ipecacuanha
For a 'noisy' cough in children.

Lachesis
For those who wake up grumpy.

Laurocerasus
For emphysema.

Ledum
For glaucoma.

Lycopodium
Cures a craving for sweet foods. Also for insomnia.

Natrum muriaticum
For the backward child, for a craving for salt, migraine, guilty feelings and depression.

Nitric acid
For curing a craving for fatty food. Also for piles.

Nux vomica
For the sort of cold that starts with a sore spot inside the nose, and the lumbago which is worse in dry weather.

Opium
For strokes.

Phosphorus
For depression in intelligent people.

Pulsatilla
For catarrh, allergy, sneezing, bedwetting, single joint rheumatism.

Rhus toxicodendron
For rheumatism.

Ruta
For painful knees, or for failing vision.

Sanguinaria
For painful shoulder.

Sepia
For menopausal symptoms, palpitations, warts and the 'always tired'.

Silica
For rough hands, skin problems, migraine.

Sulphur
For itchy skin problems and for piles.

Tellurium
For osteoarthritis in the neck or spine.

Thuja
For bedwetting.

Valeriana
For anxiety, mood swing or insomnia.

This short list of symptomatic homoeopathic remedies will probably only be effective if used in conjunction with your constitutional remedy reached through a homoeopathic consultation.

IODINE

MINERALS do not figure so very prominently on the shelves of health-food shops, which is curious in a way, because it was a mineral – elemental iodine – that was one of the very first modern health foods!

Iodine-deficiency goitre used to be so common in the Pennines that it was called 'Derbyshire neck'. In what used to be Yugoslavia there were thought to be 1.5 million victims, and in parts of the Indian sub-continent 90 per cent of the population have iodine-deficiency goitre. Over 20 years ago the British Ministry of Health accepted the principle of iodine-fortified table salt, and iodine-lack goitres are rare in Britain today, iodine having become a health food without our noticing it.

The body contains 20 – 30mg of iodine, most of which is in the thyroid gland, though the blood and tissues contain minute amounts of the element.

The thyroid relies on iodine to produce its hormone, and when this is missing from the diet, the gland swells as it tries to make more of the hormone in the absence of dietary iodine. This swelling is a goitre and, large or small, its treatment is a purely medical matter. Although once very prevalent in the West, goitres have now been virtually eradicated.

Goitre is the commonest symptom of iodine deficiency, but a severe lack during pregnancy and early childhood can cause cretinism (a condition present from birth characterised by dwarfism and mental retardation).

That we need so little iodine to keep us fit and well should alert us to the fact that 'small' can be important in the matter of nutritional health.

There is a lot of current interest in the iodine which appears in the fall-out when nuclear reactors explode. Then, if the thyroid gland is in any way deficient in iodine, a radioactive form 'homes in' on the thyroid where it can produce thyroid cancer. To counter this, potassium iodide was issued to fall-out victims when the Russian nuclear power plant at Chernobyl exploded some years ago.

Do You Need Supplementation?

There are substances called goitrogens present in the diet and sometimes in water supplies, and these interfere with iodine absorption. The commonest goitrogens occur in plants of the brassica family (cabbage, turnips, etc.). Excessive doses of cobalt and manganese are also liable to interfere with iodine absorption. Women are more susceptible to iodine lack than are men, and in puberty and pregnancy adequate intakes of iodine are important if goitres are to be avoided.

— FOOD SOURCES —

Most foods contain little or no iodine, the main exceptions being milk, sea fish and other seafoods.

Due to our relatively high salt intake, most of us get more than enough iodine. Those on low-salt or salt-free diets will find that fish, liver, eggs, wholemeal bread and dairy produce provide adequate intake. Iodised products other than kelp do not feature prominently in the health-food market.

Seaweeds such as kelp and carrageen (Irish moss) provide adequate 'green' sources of supplementary iodine, as does milk.

Dosage, Incompatibilities and Toxicity

Iodine salts ingested in a natural way should provide 140µg per day to prevent goitre. Excessive intake over 1 000µg (1mg) per day is toxic and can cause thyroid overactivity.

Interaction with goitrogens (see page 67), cobalt and manganese occurs.

An excessive intake of iodine – usually contained in an iodine-rich cough mixture – can produce or aggravate acne. Seaweed eaters (mostly Japanese) run a risk of taking too much iodine. They also develop toxic goitres – and sometimes acne.

GOOD BUYS

Any kelp product (available in tablet form in the health food shop). See the Pharmafax.

See also: **Goitre.**

IRON

THE mineral iron is the most vital component of our red blood cells – all 20,000 billion of them – and yet our whole body contains only 3.5 – 4.5g of it, the amount of iron in a fair-sized builder's nail. (This is a prime example of little in weight being 'weighty' in health terms.) The reason you need so little iron is due to a miracle of biological conservation, and a feat of recycling that the most sophisticated man-made recycling plant can in no way match.

Once it has been absorbed, iron tends to be efficiently stored – in fact, these stores can account for 30 per cent of the total body iron. Your body is very miserly with its use of iron. Fit men lose iron mostly due to cell loss from the skin and from the bowel. Women lose much more iron during their fertile lives, through menstruation and having babies.

The body regulates its internal mineral iron by an incredibly sensitive and selective absorption process. Normally we absorb about 6–10 per cent of the iron in our food, but if you get anaemic you can absorb up to 60 per cent. Certain other nutritional factors alter iron absorption – Vitamin C enhances absorption, while tea and coffee drinking inhibits it. Nobody understands how the absorption organ knows how much iron to absorb to keep the balance *right*. But it does almost all of the time.

Signs and Symptoms of Deficiency

These are listed in the section on Anaemia on page 175.

Do You Need Supplementation?

Children under five and women in their fertile years probably do. Teenage males need almost as much iron as do females because of unpredictable growth spurts.

Pregnancy is a time when women need to look carefully at their iron intake, especially if their personal tastes or preferences do not include good daily helpings of iron-rich food. During pregnancy, and for three months after the baby is born, a 30–60mg supplement is required. Larger doses are necessary if the iron supplement also contains calcium carbonate, as this inhibits iron absorption.

— FOOD SOURCES —

Generous quantities of meat, poultry and fish, together with Vitamin C-rich foods ensure iron equilibrium in most cases, but vegetarians should eat kelp, brewer's yeast, blackstrap molasses, wheatgerm, raisins and beet. Some cereal foods are iron-fortified.

Iron-rich Food
Meat, including liver; dried fruits; dark green vegetables; sardines; prunes; whole-grain cereals; eggs. Cooking in iron pots increases the iron content of food.

ANAEMIA AND IRON

Iron-deficiency anaemia is the commonest mineral deficiency disease. Deficiency is particularly common in children in groups where late weaning is combined with inappropriate feeding. Some 28 per cent of children of Asian origin in Bradford were recently found to be anaemic, as were up to 27 per cent of similar children in Birmingham (where, incidentally, 18 per cent of children of *European* origin are anaemic). US Health and Nutrition studies have demonstrated that 95 per cent of children between the ages of one and five, and most women during their fertile years, have an intake of iron below the RNI (Reference Nutrient Intake) of 11.3mg per day.

Tiredness and fatigue are major symptoms of anaemia. The physical work of 75 women, as measured by a treadmill performance, was examined. The group consisted of women who were either anaemic or had normal blood counts and haemoglobin levels. Those who were not anaemic could perform well under the severest treadmill settings selected. Anaemic women could only stay on the treadmill for a comparatively short time before becoming exhausted. Clearly iron supplements, perhaps augmented with Vitamin C, are indicated in the tiredness of anaemia.

The management of iron-deficiency anaemia is basically a medical problem. It is possible to improve iron nutrition by means of suitable diet manipulation, but in most cases iron supplements are necessary.

COLDS AND IRON

Iron deficiency has been shown to impair the immune response, so children and elderly people can be frequent victims of simple infections such as colds, and may well benefit from iron supplements.

A tonic containing a cocktail of vitamins and iron is marketed as Minadex, and many mothers swear by it as a cure for recurrent colds in toddlers.

HAIR PROBLEMS AND IRON

Iron deficiency has often been associated with hair loss, so it would make sense to supplement with iron if falling hair or alopecia is a problem.

MENORRHAGIA AND IRON

Both young and pre-menopausal women who suffer from menorrhagia, or heavy periods, respond well to iron supplementation. Sometimes, however, iron supplements make heavy periods heavier, in which case medical advice should be sought.

TIREDNESS, FATIGUE AND IRON

See Anaemia and Iron above.

IRON APATHY

Iron has traditionally been looked upon as a tonic, but this attitude towards this important mineral has been somewhat diluted by an increased level of medical knowledge of the anaemias. That iron may still possess unexpected health bonuses has been suggested by research at the University of North Dakota that related iron status to the cognitive performance (intake of knowledge) of healthy university students. Iron status (stored iron) was shown to be significantly related to cognitive performance and verbal fluency, attention span and the ability to concentrate.

Work carried out at the University of Colorado has linked mild iron deficiency in three- to six-year-old children with reversible alterations in cognitive function. This iron apathy is more pronounced when the anaemia is long-standing. Sometimes the classic signs and symptoms of anaemia can be experienced, and yet a blood test confirms a normal haemoglobin level. This puzzles doctors. Such people may have low iron stores and a low serum iron level (iron is present in blood cells and in the serum in which they circulate – sometimes in differing levels).

Dosages, Toxicity and Side Effects

Dosage varies with the preparation – a meaningful iron supplement would contain 12mg of iron in conjunction with 30mg of Vitamin C.

High intakes are dangerous for the small number of haemochromatosis sufferers, who should on no account take iron preparations of any sort. This condition cannot be controlled just by reducing dietary iron, because once iron is stored extensively it can be toxic when deposited in tissues not designed by nature as iron stores.

Dietary Reference Values for Iron, mg per day

Age	LRNI		EAR		RNI	
	Males	Females	Males	Females	Males	Females
11–18 yr	6.1	8.0	8.7	11.4	11.3	14.8
19–49 yr	8.7	8.0	6.7	11.4	8.7	14.8
50+ yr	4.7	4.7	6.7	6.7	8.7	8.7

Iron therapy is associated with side effects in many people. These include gastrointestinal irritation (nausea, vomiting), diarrhoea or constipation. Sometimes these are so severe that injection therapy has to be considered. Often, however, by changing the iron preparation or reducing the dose, it is possible to gradually promote iron absorption without too much in the way of adverse reaction.

Incompatibility

Iron absorption is decreased by many antacid preparations, by some antibiotics (tetracyclines), by phosphates in soft drinks and by substances called phytates found in bran or fibre. (Here we can see a health food *aggravating* a health problem, although some people who cannot tolerate fibre-rich diets because of 'gas bloating' in the bowel find that iron supplements cure this fibre incompatibility.)

Iron supplementation is known to interfere with the absorption of zinc, and those on long-term supplementation need to consider concurrent zinc supplementation.

GOOD BUYS

The preparations most popularly sold in chemists are limited to sales in pharmacies as opposed to health-food outlets. If, as seems reasonable, symptom-free absorption is unrelated to tablet formulation it would seem justifiable to advise the most economical product as the best. NHS ferrous iron preparations like Feospan Spansule (Smith Kline Beecham), Fergon (Sterling Winthrop) and Ferrocap (Consolidated Chemical) are all competitively priced. Fersaday (Evans) produce a very economical one-a-day iron supplement which falls into the *Best Buy* category.

Iron can be present in health foods in different forms. If a product says it contains elemental iron, it means the iron is in the form of a simple salt such as iron sulphate. The advantage of this is that it gives an easy index of how much iron is being swallowed. But many would say that less simple forms (e.g. iron succinates) are better absorbed if less easy to evaluate pharmacologically. This is an age-old running debate that is set to continue.

Synergistic Iron (QUEST)
This formula contains 25mg of elemental iron dose plus a blend of other vitamins and minerals to aid absorption. A process of amino acid chelation using rice protein has been used which claims to enhance absorption and lessen any allergic reactions.

Blackstrap Molasses Iron (FOOD SUPPLEMENT COMPANY)
A combination of blackstrap molasses and extra iron with added Vitamin C to aid absorption. One capsule per day provides approximately 15mg of iron (i.e. the top end of the DRV scale, see the table, page 72). This formula is designed to be kind to the stomach.

Other commonly available iron supplements are listed in the Pharmafax.

See also: **Anaemia; Balding and Scalp Hair Problems; Colds; Immunodepression; Menorrhagia; Tiredness and Fatigue.**

MAGNESIUM

THERE is not an enormous amount of magnesium in the human body – about 25g (1oz) to be precise. It is an essential part of many of the body's enzyme systems, and is present in the cells of all the tissues. However, about 70 per cent of that ounce of magnesium resides in our bones and teeth, where it appears to be well locked in. A limited amount of magnesium is therefore on call to the rest of the body, which suggests that we rely very much on a *regular day-to-day* intake of the element to make sure that our needs are well and truly met.

Signs and Symptoms of Deficiency

It is extremely difficult to pin down magnesium deficiency, even using quite sophisticated procedures like blood and urine testing. As a result the medical profession tends to see our bodies as so very efficient at self-regulating magnesium content that, for all intents and purposes, magnesium deficiency just does not exist, except in very rare circumstances!

However, magnesium deficiency symptoms may include loss of appetite, palpitations, irritability, weakness, insomnia, muscle tremor, numbness and tingling sensations, confusion, personality change and skin problems. Magnesium deficiency can be *brought about* by many disorders – diarrhoea and vomiting, for instance – some of which are outlined in the pages following.

— FOOD SOURCES—

The RNI (Reference Nutrient Intake) for magnesium is around 300mg per day (slightly less for women), but the average intake is very much less.

The most common magnesium-rich foods include cocoa or chocolate (plain chocolate more than milk); nuts (especially cashews, almonds and Brazils) – but you have to eat close on 100g (4oz) per day to get your RNI, and that's a lot of nuts for most people; and seafood (especially winkles, whelks and shrimps) – but who eats masses of these?

Foods of vegetable origin are important sources. Magnesium is an essential component of chlorophyll (involved in plant photosynthesis) and some vegetables are particularly rich, such as beans, peas and spinach beet.

All grain is a good source (especially barley and wheat).

But a diet is, of course, a mixed thing, and the general foodstuffs we tend to eat regularly *in quantity* are very poor providers of magnesium. Meat and fish contain only relatively small quantities, and the same is true of fruits, salads and dairy products.

It has been calculated that about 12 per cent of our daily intake of magnesium *can be* derived from water, and that if you live in a hard-water area you can get 18 per cent via your water supply.

Do You Need Supplementation?

Those who are overweight and decide to slim by opting for a high-protein, low-carbohydrate diet are self-selecting a really low-magnesium diet. Those who exist on an 'institutional' diet for a long time can suffer as nutritional stores of the mineral become depleted.

Dr Jean Durlach, author of the most modern textbook on magnesium, is on record as saying 'Dietary magnesium in many regions, and particularly in France, appears to be insufficient to satisfy any daily need.' This opinion was echoed by many delegates from various countries attending the Fifth International Magnesium Symposium in Kyoto, Japan, recently. They heard their president report that 'New food habits in Japanese people living in urban areas and in the younger generation, induce an impressive decrease in the magnesium/calcium ratio in their daily food.' The president also went on to encourage the use of magnesium supplements by expectant mothers, and those taking the diuretics or beta-blocker drugs most commonly prescribed for high blood pressure and/or heart failure.

All in all, the consensus of nutritional opinion is that the magnesium supplied by the average diet is at best only marginal. All sorts of things are liable to tip the balance the wrong way and produce magnesium-lack symptomatology. It could be the sort of bread you eat, whether or not you do a heavy job or play an exhausting game that makes you sweat a lot, which is important in this context. Men tend to get depleted of magnesium more easily than women. Genetic factors may decide how efficient or otherwise your absorption organ is at leaching out the magnesium from foods. Where you live (magnesium content of soil, for instance) and the hardness of your water supply is also important.

So it rather looks as though whenever and wherever you look for evidence of magnesium deficiency in the diet you tend to find it. Women can suffer as well as men. A recent survey of pregnant women from a wide sweep of economic backgrounds showed that their magnesium intake varied from 103–333mg per day (the RNI intake is in excess of 270mg per day for a pregnant woman). Another group of doctors writing in the *American Journal of Clinical Nutrition* carried out meticulous 7-day metabolic balance studies on a group of healthy white women in Tennessee and found that their mean daily magnesium intakes were only 60 per cent of the recommended intake. It is highly likely that a similar state of affairs operates elsewhere in the world.

Incompatibilities and Interactions

In the USA there have been magnesium watchers around since the 1930s, and they have recorded, according to Dr Mildred Seelig of the Goldwater Memorial Hospital, New York University Medical Center, a gradual fall-off in the magnesium content of the national diet over the years. One interesting fact about magnesium is that certain nutrients and foods *increase* the body's *requirements* of magnesium. Vitamin D and phosphates fall into this category. This provides us with an insight on new ways of becoming magnesium deficient.

There was a sharp rise in all our intakes of Vitamin D in the 1940s and 1950s which came about by the fortification of various foods, especially margarine, with Vitamin D. Shortly after this, there was an expansion in the soft drinks industry on both sides of the Atlantic. The consumption of soft drinks provides us with a major and unexpected source of phosphates in our diets (which inhibit absorption of magnesium), and the volume of consumption of these soft drinks has been rising rapidly for the last quarter of a century. (Incidentally, while zero-calorie soft drinks are good for slimming, caffeine-rich soft drinks are not good for children, and sugar-rich soft drinks are not good for teeth or obesity.)

And so we have a very interesting and maybe worrying situation in which, not only are we eating *less* magnesium, but we are also eating much *more* in the way of foods and drinks that demand *more* magnesium to keep us well topped up with this vital element.

Our children are likely to be in jeopardy too. Some 30 years ago, the British Paediatric Association pointed out how much more Vitamin D we were giving our children each day – especially if we unconsciously add to it with a diet supplement. For instance, a toddler taking 1 litre (1¾ pints) of dried milk per day together with 25g (1oz) of cereal and a teaspoonful of cod liver oil could tot up a daily total of over 4,000 iu of Vitamin D daily – far more than is necessary to protect him or her from rickets and enough perhaps to point the child in the direction of the magnesium deficiency syndromes.

The magnesium intake of young people has recently caused concern to the American Dietary Association, which looked at what students ate and drank in 50 colleges in the USA. It was a huge task, and the findings were quite worrying from the point of view of magnesium intake, which averaged only a mean of 250mg per day (suggested RNI is 300mg for a 15- to 18-year-old). What made the position more worrying was that the phosphorus:magnesium ratio was 7:1. This is a high ratio when one remembers that phosphorus is a phosphate, and means that the more phosphorus you take, the more magnesium you need to keep your magnesium topped up.

Another cause for concern as far as magnesium deficiency is concerned is that nowadays everybody is tending to eat much more fibre. In many ways this is an excellent health trend, but high-fibre foods – brown bread, brown rice, oatmeal, muesli, or phytate-enriched white bread – all tend to reduce magnesium absorption. Intake of fibre should be matched by extra magnesium intake.

A high calcium intake may lower magnesium absorption. This is particularly relevant to disorders and diseases of the bone (see pages 80 and 272).

ALCOHOL INTAKE AND MAGNESIUM

A change of lifestyle most Western countries demonstrate these days is an increasing intake of alcohol by both young and old. It has been amply demonstrated that even moderate social drinking is what nutritionalists call *magnesuretic*. In other words, more magnesium is pumped out of the body through the kidneys, and causes (magnesium-lack) palpitations. Just one extra alcoholic drink can force that little bit of magnesium out of the tissue fluids and into the urine to put some drinkers out of magnesium balance for a while: their heart registers its complaint by over-active palpitations for an hour or so.

The palpitations suffered by alcoholics who are 'drying out' can also be associated with low blood magnesium.

CARDIAC PROBLEMS AND MAGNESIUM

Healthy hearts need good magnesium stores, for magnesium is a major element in one of the heart's three principal nutrients (see page 202). This has gradually been recognised over the years by orthodox medicine.

In the late 1960s surgeons began to operate on the heart much more commonly to repair of all sorts of cardiac abnormalities. To do so they used what is called a heart-lung machine to take over the function of the patient's heart during cardiac surgery, often for considerable periods. In some cases, once the surgery was over, the heart seemed to have trouble starting to beat regularly and efficiently again on its own. Eventually it was found that in such patients low serum magnesium levels occurred. Subsequently it was decided to add extra magnesium to the pump system and the problem was rectified. Later, in the 1970s, when open-heart surgery was becoming commonplace, surgeons started to give intravenous doses of magnesium to their patients routinely, and the troublesome irregularity of the pulse of patients post-operatively became very rare indeed.

Magnesium has also been used quite extensively recently in the management of heart attacks, especially at a time when there was a vogue for the use of anticoagulants in such cases. In one study, out of a series of 100 heart-attack patients who were given magnesium therapy, only one died, compared with 60 out of 200 similar patients who were treated solely with anti-coagulants.

A report in *The Times* recently concerned experiments conducted at the Los Angeles County University of Southern California Medical Center. Using the method of atomic absorption spectrophotometry, as an estimate of magnesium status in 103 patients who had been admitted to a coronary-care unit, researchers found that in no less than 53 per cent of cases an abnormally low magnesium status was demonstrable. Dr Robert Rude, one of the specialists involved in the study, emphasised the link between cardiac arrhythmias and magnesium deficiency, and divulged that magnesium-deficient heart patients at the University Medical School's Cardiology Division were being given regular magnesium supplements. This practice is slowly becoming an everyday practice on a worldwide basis.

DYSMENORRHOEA AND MAGNESIUM

Magnesium and pyridoxine therapy has been shown to benefit the pains and cramps of dysmenorrhoea.

KIDNEY STONES AND MAGNESIUM

Research in the USA has shown a close connection between a low-magnesium diet and the formation of stones in the kidneys. The magnesium deficiency can be brought about by crops grown in soils with a low magnesium content (and which have been fertilised artificially) or by drinking soft water (much less rich in magnesium than hard).

Today the numbers of recurrent stone sufferers whose disease has been virtually abolished by the therapeutic use of magnesium runs into thousands.

It seems highly likely that, in the interests of keeping well away from the terror of kidney stones, particular attention should be paid to the maintenance of an adequate magnesium intake. The supplement could include Vitamin B_6 as well, which is also earning itself an enviable reputation in the field of renal health.

OSTEOPOROSIS AND MAGNESIUM

The bones are a major depository of the body's magnesium, and if there is a blood or tissue deficiency of the mineral, the bones may be leached and become less healthy. There is a great deal of research concerning magnesium and the bone disease of osteoporosis, and that there is a beneficial connection cannot be denied.

PMS AND MAGNESIUM

One of the most interesting studies on the subject of PMS (Pre-Menstrual Syndrome) has recently been carried out by a group of doctors from the Royal Sussex County Hospital in Brighton. This was stimulated by research carried out in the USA by Dr G.E. Abraham, who had first suggested that many of the diverse symptoms of PMS might be due to magnesium deficiency.

A survey involving the women members of 50 colleges in the USA showed that the food which they ate provided only sub-optimal levels of magnesium. Women need at least 270mg of magnesium per day to maintain themselves in magnesium balance, yet the magnesium taken by the average female studied in this survey averaged out at only 204mg per day.

Dr Mildred Seelig, the American magnesium expert, feels that the low magnesium status of women is liable to be eroded even more by the current interest in fibre and dieting. The increase in fibre is fair enough from the slimming point of view, but fibre-rich foods tend relentlessly to reduce magnesium absorption.

Magnesium supplementation has been shown to be helpful in some forms of PMS (see page 282).

TIREDNESS, FATIGUE AND MAGNESIUM

Trials have shown that magnesium can help alleviate chronic tiredness, loss of appetite, apathy, weakness and muscular uncoordination.

Dosage

A meaningful dietary supplement would be 100–300mg per day.

Dietary Reference Values for Magnesium, mg per day

Age	EAR	
	Males	Females
19 + yr	250	200

Additional amounts to be added to pre-pregnancy DRVs
Lactating women + 50

GOOD BUYS

Magnesium-OK (WASSEN)
A very good formulation, backed by research. Each daily-dose tablet contains 145mg of magnesium plus other minerals and vitamins.

Synergistic Magnesium (QUEST)
150mg of magnesium combined with calcium, Vitamin B$_6$ and phosphorus. Quest have also used an amino acid process of chelation to enhance absorption. The amino acids have been derived from rice protein to avoid any allergic reactions. This could be particularly helpful for kidney stone problems.

Aminochel Magnesium (HEALTHCRAFTS)
See also: **Alcoholism; Cardiac Problems; Dysmenorrhoea; Kidney Stones; Osteoporosis; PMS; Tiredness and Fatigue.**

MARINE OILS

As with plant oils, there has been a surge of interest in the essiential fatty acids marine oils contain. Their importance to the prostaglandins is discussed under that head in the Glossary, as is that of the essential fatty acids themselves, from which the prostaglandins are synthesised.

The British nutritional scientist Hugh Sinclair became interested in marine oils in the 1930s, and it was he who first put forward the theory that it was the type of fat (oils) that Eskimos consumed as part of their everyday diet that protected them against thrombosis diseases, diseases to which the rest of the world is very prone. Later in the 1970s, he subjected himself to an Eskimo diet – a diet very rich in seal meat, which is, like cod liver oil, very rich in certain essential fatty acids that are nature's precursors to the prostaglandins. While on this diet, Sinclair noted that if he cut himself shaving then his face bled rather a lot. He suspected that his 'blood-clotting time' had been altered by his diet, and he confirmed this by means of a simple blood test. Thus the concept of a dietary method of managing the major disease that our flesh is heir to was first made manifest.

Marine oils, particularly cod liver oil, are rich in essential fatty acids which are valuable in the treatment of the blood-clotting diseases. They are also helpful in the treatment of rheumatism, artery problems, problems of the gall bladder and the prevention of heart disease.

Dosage, Contraindications and Side Effects

Dosage depends on how much fish you regularly eat. If you have an ounce or more daily of the oily fish – mackerel, sardine or salmon – you need no routine supplementation. For once-a-week oily fish eaters, one 5ml teaspoon of cod liver oil should be taken on non-fish days. For non-oily fish eaters, 5ml daily is a reasonable dose.

Cod liver oil and other marine oils should not be taken by anyone known to have a bleeding disorder – haemophilia or recurrent nosebleeds – and should not be taken in conjunction with anti-coagulant therapy. It is inadvisable to take marine oils when undergoing dental treatment involving extraction.

Reported adverse reactions are occasional nausea and belching.

GOOD BUYS

There are several marine oils available in health food shops, some made from fish liver (cod and other fish, for instance), some from whole fish. Some are concentrated blends of fish oils.

Cod liver oil, pure, and from a reputable manufacturer, is the best to buy (see Cod Liver Oil).

MAXEPA (NOVEX)

This is a marine oil product developed by the cod liver oil

industry which contains Omega 3 triglycerides in each capsule in the following proportions: eicosapentaenoic acid 180mg, and docosahexaenoic acid 120mg. Five such capsules per day is the advised dose. It is often thought of as a 'super' cod liver oil, and is prescribable under the NHS.

Pulse (SEVEN SEAS)
Rich in Omega 3 marine triglycerides. Each capsule contains 500mg of pure fish body oil, natural Vitamin E, and a gelatin/glycerine shell. It contains no synthetic drugs, no artificial colours, no preservatives, and is also sugar-free.

Lanes Range
Lanepa 1,000mg capsules contain concentrated fish body oils, and natural Vitamin E as an antioxidant. The capsule shell is gelatin/glycerine. It contains no preservatives, sugar, starch, added flavours or colours.

Fish Oil Liquid contains 150ml of liquid concentrated fish oil per dose with a natural lemon flavour, and natural Vitamin E as an antioxidant. This product contains no gluten, artificial flavours or preservatives.

Omega-3 Fish Oil (WASSEN)
This is an extra-concentrated blend of marine lipids in a small capsule for easy swallowing. It is also salt-free, and contains Vitamin E as an antioxidant.

Epopa (VITALIA)
A mixed plant oil and fish oil product.

Halibut Liver Oil (HEALTHILIFE, BOOTS)
Each capsule provides pure halibut liver oil and soya oil. The shell is gelatin/glycerine. The recommended dose is one capsule daily, which provides 4,000 iu of Vitamin A. (See warning on page 85.)

> **— CAUTION —**
>
> Halibut liver oil poses a possible overdosage hazard. The halibut liver oil story is complex. To start with, sources vary widely with regard to the content of Vitamins A and D, but some samples are very rich in A. Hypervitaminosis has occurred when people overdose with halibut liver oil. It is virtually impossible to overdose with cod liver oil or other marine oils. The small amount of marine oil in the daily dose of halibut liver oil makes a very small contribution to cardio-vasculor health.

See also: **Cod Liver Oil; Glossary; Plant Oils; Artery Problems; Arthritis and Rheumatism; Balding and Scalp Hair Problems; Cardiac Problems; Gall Bladder Problems; Hypertension; Rickets.**

PLANT OILS

TODAY there is an explosion of interest among both doctors and nutritionists in essential fatty acids in general, and gamma linolenic acid (GLA) in particular. The importance of these to the health of the prostaglandins is discussed under that heading in the Glossary, as is that of the essential fatty acids from which the prostaglandins are also synthesised.

The GLA of evening primrose oil is the most effective and potent, but GLA is present in and can be extracted from a wide variety of plants and their seeds, for instance borage and linseed. It has been claimed, however, that the GLA of borage, linseed and other plant oils is not so freely available as that in evening primrose oils.

Plant oils containing good quantities of GLA are useful for general well-being and skin health, and in the treatment of skin conditions, artery problems, rheumatism, fibrocystic breast disease, hyperkinesis, multiple sclerosis and PMT.

Dosage, Contraindications and Side Effects

There are no EAR, RNI, LRNI or RDA values for plant oil products. In the absence of such official guidelines, doses are best and most safely met by taking 1,000 iu of the plant oil daily, or if the product is sold as a concentrate then a safe dose would be 160–240mg of linolenic acid twice daily.

If GLA products are to be taken for gynaecological symptoms, the presence of gynaecological cancer should first be excluded by a doctor.

Schizophrenics should not take GLA products except under medical supervision, and neither should epileptics nor those who are predisposed to fits or are taking drugs to prevent fits (your doctor or pharmacist will advise).

No major adverse reactions have been reported. Some takers complain of nausea, indigestion and headaches.

GOOD BUYS

Apart from the pre-eminence of evening primrose oil, it is difficult to find convincing scientific evidence on which to base a best-buy policy with reference to GLA enrichment products, which are on the whole competitively priced and of a high standard.

Glanolin 250 and 500 (LANES)
These products contain an oil obtained from blackcurrant seeds. They also contain a relatively high percentage of GLA per capsule, which means that fewer capsules need to be taken, an advantage for those who have difficulty swallowing.

Galanol Range (LIFEPLAN)
These products use mainly oil of borage seeds (as well as evening primrose oil), and also contain high amounts of GLA. Again the benefits of large amounts of GLA mean that fewer capsules need to be taken to give an equivalent GLA intake.

Galanol Gold capsules contain a blend of oil of borage seeds, evening primrose oil and Vitamin E in a gelatin/glycerine capsule, to give a GLA content of 16 per cent.

Super Galanol capsules contain oil of borage seeds (or starflower oil) and Vitamin E; the GLA content is between 25 and 27 per cent per capsule. This is extremely high, and as a result the recommended number of capsules that need to be taken is reduced.

Sunflower (or Safflower) Oil Capsules (HEALTHILIFE)
These contain 500mg of pure sunflower seed oil (or safflower seed oil) in a gelatin/glycerine shell. They contain no additives, preservatives or allergens.

Pure Linseed Oil (G & G)
This is a high quality linseed oil. It is cold-pressed and unrefined-so it retains all the beneficial qualities of the linseeds. It contains no gluten, grains, lactose, sugar, colouring or yeast.

Starflower Oil (ROCHE)
This is a high-GLA product.

NHS PRESCRIPTION REMEDIES

Some GLA products, marketed by Searle, are available on UK NHS prescription.

Efamast – 3–4 capsules per day (to be taken for 8–12 weeks).

Epogam – For adult eczema in capsule form: 2 twice daily (for 8–12 weeks).

Epogram Paediatric – For children over one year, 2 snip-off capsules for squeezing onto food daily.

See also: **Glossary; Evening Primrose Oil; Artery Problems; Arthritis and Rheumatism; Fibrocystic Breast Disease; Hyperkinesis; MS; PMS.**

POLLEN, PROPOLIS AND ROYAL JELLY

ALL too often in the past, orthodox medicine has stumbled badly in its rejection of certain useful medicaments because strictly honourable and scientifically-orientated medical practitioners just couldn't understand *how* the various substances that appeared to be therapeutic to the patients who swallowed them, could possibly 'work'. The marine oils were for years an example of this attitude, and three other substances – pollen products, propolis and royal jelly – fall to some extent into a similar category. Although not having much in the way of scientific evidence, these products do have a degree of support which makes them worth considering. It is perhaps rather odd that a creature from the insect world is involved in all three.

POLLEN

Pollen is the fine, granular substance produced by the anthers of flowers which fundamentally contains the male reproductive element of plants. Pollens come in all shapes and sizes, ranging from one-tenth of an inch to a fraction of a micron in length. Some are powdery and some are sticky, depending upon whether wind or insects are involved in the plant's reproductive cycle. Pollen enters our food chain mostly through the consumption of honey and it is often forgotten that honey has been a staple item of diet for many thousands of years. The plant world produces prodigious amounts of pollen (the spruce forests of Sweden alone are said to produce some 75,000 tons of pollen a year).

Pollen, when analysed chemically, is disclosed to be a complex of more than 20 amino acids (protein building-blocks) together with 7 vitamins and various sugars, saturated and unsaturated fats, and 17 minerals and micronutrients.

Whether or not the natural nutrients in pollen become part and parcel of commercial honey depends on the manufacturing process that occurs between the honeycomb in the hive and the honey on your plate. Fine filtration and heat treatments tend to combine in many cases to convert what appears to be one of Nature's super-foods into just another calorie-rich sweetener.

Do You Need Pollen?

You might consider it worthwhile in four specific situations.

INFLUENZA AND POLLEN

The few published trials which provide evidence of scientific value for pollen therapy are not very impressive. One fairly large trial involving 510 employees of a Swedish industrial company sought to establish whether or not a pollen extract (Fluaxin) would influence sickness rates (time off work) during an influenza epidemic. When the trial was concluded Fluaxin was considered to demonstrate the efficacy of the product because 98 per cent of employees taking Fluaxin had stayed at work during an epidemic. But the Fluaxin tablets contained, as well as pollen, 100mg of aspirin, and aspirin is well-known to be effective in controlling the symptomatology of influenza and similar illnesses. Any scientific conclusion to this study would seem to be extremely problematical.

PROSTATITIS AND POLLEN

Prostatitis is a relatively common condition (see page 285), and can occur in various forms, but it usually responds promptly to orthodox medical treatment. It may be associated with enlargement of the prostate gland, in which case it is less easy to manage. On theoretical grounds it is difficult to see how the complex of amino acids and vitamins that constitute the substance of pollen could have an effect on prostatitis, but uncontrolled honey trials in Scandinavia (one involving 12 cases and another 172) claimed an excellent clear-up rate in prostatitis patients (*The Healing Power of Pollen*, Thorsons, 1989). And recent research involving Cernilton, a rye grass pollen extract, has shown such significant results that it has become a Gold Standard therapy.

GENERAL DEBILITY IN THE ELDERLY AND POLLEN

It is interesting, perhaps, that one of the few double blind trials involving pollen (the sort of trial that impresses doctors) took place with reference to a disease that is very difficult to define, but easy enough to recognise clinically. This is a condition in which the victim tires easily, has a poor appetite and a tendency to weariness, apathy and listlessness, together with an abdication of the general business of everyday living.

A consultant to the French Ministry of Social Affairs carried out a double blind trial of pollen tablets which involved two groups of 48 men in their early seventies, who were considered to be suffering from 'general debility of the elderly'. Responses that were judged to be very good occurred after four weeks' therapy in 54 per cent of those taking pollen, compared to 12 per cent in those found to be taking dummy capsules. The tests used in the assessment of these patients involved measurements of strength, concentration and speed of performance of various tasks. A substantial weight gain in the pollen takers occurred during therapy. Although this trial is a small one and criteria for admission into the trial appear rather vague, the positive results seem to cry out for further assessment of pollen products in this field.

RADIATION SICKNESS AND POLLEN

Radiotherapy plays an increasingly large role in the management of malignant disease. Quite often radiotherapy is complicated by the particularly unpleasant side effects known as radiation sickness. Often this taxes the expertise of those involved in case management, and as a result there has been an increased excursion into what many doctors would consider to be fringe medicine in an attempt to mitigate radiation sickness (recently acupuncture has found considerable favour). But, back in the 1970s, the University Radiological Institute of Sarajevo used Melbrosin, a pollen capsule, in a single blind trial involving 90 patients undergoing radiotherapy. The majority of patients who took the pollen-containing treatment reported good results and suffered less sickness after their irradiation than did those taking dummy tablets.

PERFORMANCE IN SPORT AND POLLEN

Pollen is perhaps closer to a food than a medicine (this may also be said for many of the preparations found in this book). It is fashionable and profitable for athletes to be seen promoting certain foodstuffs, and in some cases sponsorship has extended into the health food market, and particularly the pollen market. Several Olympic athletes, and the one-time world heavyweight boxing champion, Muhammad Ali, have all sponsored pollen extracts. Whether or not this sort of endorsement provides any weight to arguments in favour of pollen as a health-giving and performance-enhancing substance must be a personal rather than scientific assessment.

PROPOLIS

Propolis is a resinous substance that bees use as an ingenious sealant in their hives, and which they collect from the bark of various resinous trees. It has been used as a medicine since biblical times. The classical herbalists used propolis as an ointment to treat inflammatory conditions.

Modern interest in propolis seems to have stemmed from the work of a Frenchman, Professor R. Chauvin, who became interested in the ways in which bee colonies remained free from bacterial infestation despite their very high population density. Eventually he established the fact that propolis is an antibacterial agent. Propolis has now been analysed, and consists of various resins and balsams mixed with beeswax, pollen and substances known as bioflavonoids, or Vitamin P. I have reviewed this interesting group of substances in some depth elsewhere (see Glossary and References).

The bioflavonoids have enjoyed a somewhat chequered history as regards their therapeutic capacity. Some years ago, the United States Food and Drug Administration sought withdrawal of all flavonoid drugs from the market, a proposal that was resisted. Nevertheless, really convincing evidence that propolis is therapeutic is hard to come by. Professor Kupnau of Hamburg University has demonstrated that propolis tablets seemed to increase resistance to influenza during epidemics at the university. Such so-called intervention trials are notoriously difficult to evaluate and are unpopular with doctors, but propolis has been shown to inhibit the growth of certain bacteria on culture plates in rather the same way as do conventional antibiotics. Authoritative bacterial research of this interesting facility does not seem to exist, but canny pharmaceutical companies throughout the world may well have dismissed its potential. And there is, of course, no guarantee that if such a trial had been made propolis would find a place in conventional therapeutics. Indeed the reverse might well be true because, as it is a naturally-occurring product, no possibility of patent rights could be claimed, and this would prevent any effective commercial exploitation on a large scale.

Do You Need Propolis?

There are two medical situations in which propolis supplementation might be helpful.

PEPTIC ULCERATION AND PROPOLIS

The medical management of peptic ulceration has been revolutionised over the last ten years, particularly as a result of the introduction of new drugs – the so-called H_2 receptor antagonists, which reduce the secretions of acid by 60 per cent over a 24-hour period and allow many peptic ulcers to heal. Such treatments have virtually ousted many of the previously favoured antacid remedies, as well as surgical treatment. Recent research has focused on a particular type of stomach trouble and peptic ulceration that does not respond to the new therapies and which seems to be associated with an infectious agent called campylobacter. Often in such cases the chronic ulcer-type dyspepsia is preceded by an attack of gastroenteritis.

Gastroenterologists prescribe orthodox medical treatments for campylobacter problems, but one of the few trials published involved the use of propolis in the treatment of 126 patients suffering from radiologically confirmed peptic ulceration. Patients were treated along traditional dietary lines but were given propolis in addition. The results of this trial were favourable and included early symptom relief. There was, however, a considerable relapse rate, and 6 per cent of patients had to discontinue propolis due to allergic reactions. Nevertheless, it must be stressed that the possibility of propolis being a bacteria-inhibiting substance and having a therapeutic role in the management of peptic ulceration is worthy of thought and consideration. We must hope that further research will make the position clearer. Meanwhile, propolis deserves to be considered in cases of dyspepsias that do not respond to standard therapy.

HERPES ZOSTER (SHINGLES) AND PROPOLIS

This is a relatively common condition, particularly in older age groups. Until comparatively recently, treatment consisted of the prescription of pain killers and local applications of soothing preparations. Medical treatment was revolutionised by the introduction of antiviral substances (Idoxine and Acyclovir). At a symposium on apo-therapy (use of bee products) held in the former Yugoslavia some years ago a method of treating shingles with a propolis tincture was discussed. In a small uncontrolled trial propolis was claimed to be strikingly effective in pain relief.

ROYAL JELLY

If readers feel that arguments in favour of the two bee products previously mentioned are a little thin, then they may well conclude that royal jelly as a health food stands in a therapeutic isolation that would be piteous were it not for the enthusiasm of those convinced of its efficacy.

From the scientific point of view we know what royal jelly is – a milky white, jelly-like substance secreted by special glands on the head of a worker bee, the function of which is to feed all bee larvae in the first few days of life and to feed the queen bee for the rest of her life – a period of four to five years. Most bee larvae develop into worker bees (drones hatch from unfertilised eggs; worker bees have a limited life-span of around 45 days).

Chemically, royal jelly is a complex mixture of water, carbo-hydrates, protein and fat, together with various vitamins and biologically commonplace substances including acetylcholine and inositol. Clearly, from the point of view of bee life history, royal jelly is an enormously important substance. But is it likely to have any importance to human metabolism?

Advocates of royal jelly stress the speed with which the queen bee reaches maturity (16 days compared with 21 days for workers) and her long life. But it is difficult to see how a substance that seems to have a maturation-stimulating property can be helpful therapeutically when the aim of the person taking the product is to experience a tonic effect, improve 'nervous control' (whatever that is) or use as an adaptogen (see Ginseng, page 49). Claims that royal jelly may act as some sort of sexual stimulant or aphrodisiac seem to be equally unsupported by science.

Do You Need Royal Jelly?

Perhaps the most convincing answer is that, whatever royal jelly does for bees it is unlikely to have any therapeutic effect on you on a simple size and dose factor alone. Bees need to produce considerable bee-sized amounts of royal jelly to feed their workers and queen in a hive situation, but it must be remembered that the fully-grown adult bee only weighs 0.0032 of an ounce (less as a larva). To feed up a queen clearly takes rather more royal jelly, but even so, the amount of royal jelly consumed by a queen during her growth period is likely to be about a hundredth of her total weight (say 0.000032 of an ounce).

Compared with a bee, a human is immensely heavy. Now if we are looking at the sort of dose necessary to have a developmental or any other effect on a human, really massive doses of royal jelly (several hivefuls it would seem) would presumably be necessary. But commercial doses of royal jelly are extremely small and, of course, quite expensive; huge and realistic human-sized doses would be enormously costly. In other words, royal jelly scientific therapeutics seems to be a non-starter, and I have been unable to find any double blind trial to support its sensible consideration.

WORTH TRYING

Pollen B (WASSEN)

HP Propolis (FOOD SUPPLEMENT COMPANY)

POTASSIUM

WE evolved as animals to eat food containing much more potassium than sodium, both minerals needed by the body. But our modern diets in fact contain more sodium than potassium, which is strange when you consider that our bodies actually contain twice as much potassium as they do sodium. The relationship between sodium and potassium in the body is worked out very much around the conservation of sodium, which, when humankind evolved, was much scarcer in food than was potassium. However, modern eating and food-processing practice has changed this potassium domination, and thus much more sodium gets into our bodies from the food we eat.

Sodium and potassium together play an important part in the transfer of electrons through the water content of the body – which is why they are sometimes called the electrolyte minerals. When this balance is upset – if too much sodium or salt is ingested, for instance – then potassium can be depleted, and water is *retained* in the body (to cope with the salt), causing tissue to swell and even creating extra tension within the blood vessels themselves. High salt intake has often been associated with high blood pressure, or hypertension, and strokes – although some people can cope better than others, see Hypertension and Potassium.

When you eat foods containing a high potassium content, you absorb about 90 per cent of the ingested potassium, but the blood level of the mineral remains constant – a remarkable feat of efficient absorption and excretion in action. However, if the potassium intake is low, the body switches to a high potassium absorption mode to try to compensate. Often it succeeds.

Signs and Symptoms of Deficiency

Although much potassium deficiency is caused by medical treatment (see below), there is increasing concern about the effects of the low potassium content of modern diets. The processed foods so many of us rely on these days are rich in sodium, which tips the sodium/potassium ratio off balance. And although potassium is plentiful in many fresh fruits and vegetables, it is almost entirely lost when food is subjected to processing, canning and freezing processes, and long-term boiling in large quantities of water.

Deficiency symptoms include abnormal tiredness, irritability, headaches, swelling of the feet and ankles, palpitations, and bone and joint pains. Severe deficiency can lead to mental depression and confusion.

Do You Need Supplementation?

First of all, certain people who are receiving medical treatment with some diuretic drugs can run into trouble through potassium loss. Diuretics encourage the excretion of urine, and are taken to avoid tissue fluids accumulating in the legs or abdomen, causing swelling and dyspepsia, or in the lungs causing coughing and breathlessness. (This can occur as a result of heart failure or hypertension, but there are, however, more benign causes for all these symptoms.) Unfortunately, many diuretic drugs cause excessive potassium loss from the body through the urine, and a disturbance of the sodium/potassium ratio, *unless* adequate potassium supplements are taken. This is orthodox therapy now, and your doctor will advise you. Happily, a new generation of potassium-sparing diuretics has been introduced recently.

Secondly, those who have been suffering from chronic diarrhoea or prolonged gastroenteritis may need supplementation with potassium as well as salt, as may those who repeatedly induce vomiting (such as sufferers from bulimia nervosa).

— FOOD SOURCES —

Kelp; blackstrap molasses; brewer's yeast. Those who eat bran receive a potassium bonus. Many of the seed products in health-food outlets (sunflower, sesame, etc.) are rich in potassium, as are most nuts and dried fruits, vegetable soups and fruit juices. (However, some shelled nuts and dried fruits are treated with sulphates, and are therefore high in sodium.)

Potatoes are probably the major vegetable source of potassium in everyday eating, provided they are not boiled. Most fresh vegetables contain varying levels of potassium, and are low in sodium. Microwave cooking preserves natural potassium. Fruits (especially apricots, bananas, blackcurrants and citrus) are good sources – eat raw or cook very lightly.

Meats contain high levels of potassium, but these are accompanied by increased levels of sodium (more if salt is used in processing).

CARDIAC PROBLEMS AND POTASSIUM

Potassium, like magnesium, is very much involved in the regulation of the heart's rhythm, and severe deficiency can lead to major disturbances. Potassium deficiency was identified as a culprit in heart rhythm disorder occurring during the Apollo 15 lunar exploration flights involving David Scott and James Irwin. By the time that Apollo 16 was launched, potassium-enriched foods were incorporated on this and all subsequent astronaut programmes, and no untoward depletion symptoms developed.

DIABETES AND POTASSIUM

Diabetics need to ensure an adequate potassium intake, as the potassium is needed for the proper use of sugars by the body. Without adequate cellular potassium the body has difficulty in converting blood sugar into glycogen, the important 'storage pack' that can be converted into glucose and energy very rapidly. In the absence of adequate potassium the blood sugar tends to rise, and this in turn stimulates a need for extra insulin to be secreted and, of course, the diabetic process is essentially one of increased insulin demand.

HYPERTENSION AND POTASSIUM

High sodium intake is sometimes associated with high blood pressure, but it would seem that not everyone is sensitive to salt in this way. A certain number of people with high blood pressure do manage to normalise theirs by adjusting their potassium/sodium intake to the sort of ratio that we were all designed to cope with. They can do so primarily by diet – fresh foodstuffs, avoidance of salt, salted and processed foods – but it is important to realise that the normalisation of high blood pressure is always a matter for the doctor rather than the patient to manage!

To influence the blood pressure by altering the sodium/potassium level in favour of potassium results in a very low-sodium diet that hypertensive patients will not tolerate on a long-term basis. These days most doctors favour the prescription of the very effective anti-hypertensive drugs rather than dietary manipulation.

BULIMIA NERVOSA AND POTASSIUM

Dietary measures to restore electrolyte (potassium and sodium) balance in the body are part of orthodox medical treatments for the condition of bulimia nervosa (see Anorexia Nervosa).

Dosage and Side Effects

The Reference Nutrient Intake suggestions recommended by the UK Department of Health are for 3,500mg daily. They also recommend reducing sodium intake by half as a general health policy. Apart from those who, for reasons of poor absorption or diet manipulation, need a potassium-rich supplement, the way to play the safe and healthy game as far as electrolyte intake is concerned is to reduce the intake of sodium. The most obvious thing is either to avoid added table salt or to cook food without salt. But salts are 'hidden' in many processed foods: canned or frozen vegetables; cured, smoked and canned meats, fish and sausages; peanut butter, potato crisps, salted nuts and crackers; canned or packaged soups; processed or Cheddar cheeses; sauerkraut; and large quantities of olives or salad cream.

Contraindications and Toxicity

Anyone undergoing steroid treatment of any kind can react in a complex way as far as the balance of their electrolytes is concerned, and should consult their doctor about sodium and potassium supplements.

Very large doses (in excess of 17g) will elevate blood potassium to dangerous levels. This can cause liver damage, and fatal cardiac dysrhythmias.

GOOD BUYS

B13 Potassium (NATURE'S OWN)
Contains 150mg of potassium in an easily absorbed form.

Potassium (NATURAL FLOW)
Hypo-allergenic, and suitable for vegetarians and Vegans. Each tablet contains 99mg of potassium.

NHS PRESCRIPTION PRODUCTS

There are several potassium supplements prescribable by doctors in the NHS.

Kay-Cee-L (GEISTLICH)

Leok (LEO)

NU-K (CONSOLIDATED)

Sando-K (SANDOS)

Slow-K (CIBA)
They contain more potassium per tablet than health food products.

See also: **Magnesium; Anorexia Nervosa; Cardiac Problems; Diabetes; Hypertension.**

SELENIUM

SELENIUM is one of the essential micronutrients, or trace elements. Its importance for health began to be recognised 30 years ago when Klaus Schwarz, a scientist at the US National Institute of Health, identified it as a 'new' nutrient. To start with, nobody could fathom how this selenium, which seemed necessary in such minute traces, could have an effect on health in general, on disease processes, and on ageing.

Then selenium was found to be vital to the body's production of a tissue enzyme called glutathione peroxidase. This enzyme holds a key position in the basic integrity of all cell chemistry. If our intake and absorption of selenium drops below certain vital levels, we cannot make enough of this vital enzyme for our cells to function effectively, and various manifestations of selenium deficiency are liable to occur, although in many cases this is an insidious process.

A better knowledge of selenium evolved in the 1970s. But

even so, the general public did not really start hearing about it until the 1980s, when Richard A. Passwater, US biochemist and expert in trace elements, published a book called *Selenium as Food and Medicine*. By this time a commercial health food product, known as Selenium-ACE, had been marketed, which proved to be a very suitable way of administering selenium as a diet supplement or health food.

In some ways there is a similarity between the selenium story and that of cod liver oil. Cod liver oil's therapeutic possibilities were first noticed not in the medical press, but in the testimonial files of its major manufacturer. Early evidence of health benefit from selenium in the UK was also mainly culled from the files of the manufacturers of Selenium-ACE. The majority of the testimonials referred to improvements that occurred in various rheumatic conditions while taking long-term selenium supplementation. But a sizeable minority of rheumatics stated that, although their rheumatism itself was not demonstrably better while taking selenium, their pain was easier to *cope* with. In other words, selenium had a psychotrophic effect. It seemed to help persuade many rheumatism sufferers to accept their pain almost as an 'old friend' and help them to come to terms with it.

It is thought likely that a selenium deficiency has, as a result of a neuro-enzyme effect, a link with certain diseases of the nervous system. It is also known to be an antioxidant, a chemical that 'mops up' the free radicals that attack tissues and are associated with the so-called degenerative diseases, for example arthritis as well as cardiovascular disease, cancer, ageing and artery 'hardening' (see Glossary). Clearly selenium is a very versatile but still under-researched nutrient.

Signs and Symptoms of Deficiency

Selenium is found in the soil, and in the foodstuffs grown in it, and whether or not you might suffer a deficiency is highlighted by modern medical geography – in other words, where you live. In the USA, research carried out by the USDA Technical Bulletin staff has produced some fascinating 'selenium maps' that indicate the highs and lows of soil selenium and, incidentally, the relationship between these areas and the incidence of certain diseases (see *Cancer and Selenium*, page 108).

In Britain, similar evidence is not available in such detail, but an interesting survey of selenium-bearing foodstuffs nationwide was carried out by scientists from the Ministry of Agriculture, Fisheries and Food (MAFF) in 1977, in conjunction with the Laboratory of the Government Chemist. Although it was not possible ultimately to give regional values for food selenium content, the study gave a good idea as to who might suffer a deficiency of selenium in the UK – which is virtually everyone. Substantial areas of Britain are known to have a low soil content of selenium. Crops grown on such soil are low in selenium.

The latest UK Dietary Reference Values suggest an intake of between 60 and 75µg of selenium per day. (Much modern scientific opinion, however, inclines to the view that at least 200µg per day should be taken to maintain optimum health, although some nutrition experts claim that around 100µg is adequate.) Although the UK Ministry of Agriculture puts the average British *intake* at 60µg per day, we know that only 55 per cent of dietary selenium is *absorbed*, so that average intake is decidedly deficient. Other countries have very low selenium intakes that give real cause of anxiety. For example New Zealand has a low intake of about 25µg per day – the soil is low in selenium — and many epidemiologists link this with the high incidence of cardiovascular disease in that country. A similar state of affairs obtains in Finland, where farmers are encouraged to use selenium-enriched fertilisers to enhance crop selenium.

When isolated groups of people are looked at with reference to their selenium intake alone (and this does not take into consideration any known variations of selenium absorption), quite worrying statistics of deficiency on a large scale do tend to emerge. When a geriatrician carrying out a selenium survey prepared a large series of (institutional) meals in the UK, and subjected them to selenium analysis, his sophisticated photofluorometric studies detected no selenium at all in most of them.

Dietary Reference Values for Selenium, μg per day

Age	LRNI	RNI
0 – 3 months	4	10
4 – 6 months	5	13
7 – 9 months	5	10
10 – 12 months	6	10
1 – 3 years	7	15
4 – 6 years	10	20
7 – 10 years	16	30
11 – 14 years	25	45
Men		
15 – 18 years	40	70
19 – 50 years	40	75
50 + years	40	75
Women		
15 – 18 years	40	60
19 – 50 years	40	60
50 + years	40	60
Pregnancy: No increment necessary	–	–
Lactation:	+ 15	+ 15

This table above is included to show how the selenium needs vary with age. One of the most interesting reports relevant to selenium deficiency involved a large blind trial in 1974, carried out in China in an area in which many children died of a form of infantile heart disease called Keshan Disease. The soil there was extremely low in selenium. This trial involved several thousand children, and proved convincingly that selenium supplementation virtually eliminated a disease which previously killed hundreds of children each year.

Selenium in Food

The list in the box opposite is adapted from published figures and gives an idea of what might be considered to be the maximum amount of selenium found in a wide variety of raw foodstuffs. Almost all cooking or reheating drastically detracts from the *real* selenium content of all of these foods, and when we actually swallow them we only absorb about half of the selenium they contain!

If we look at any food table that shows relative selenium contents it is possible to spot 'best buys'. But even so, there are pitfalls for the unwary. Fish and shellfish are a good source of selenium, and are also cardioprotective because of their marine oil content. Many authorities, however, point out that, due to the way selenium is bonded with other elemental substances in fish, only a small proportion of the selenium in fish is actually absorbed into our body. Eating more fish, therefore, although providing a health bonus in other ways, will not solve the tendency in the UK towards selenium deficiency.

Another way to get more selenium into our system would be to increase the daily intake of cereals. But here again there are potential and actual problems. The selenium in cereals is very much influenced by geography, too. The flour that is traditionally used by the bread-making industry in the UK mostly came from North American sources until recently, and has a relatively high selenium content. But the modern vogue is for 'home-baked' special breads like wholemeal, which are made from European flour. This means that much less selenium is taken in our cereal food. And other cereal sources in the UK (pastas, rice, breakfast cereals in general) are among the lowest in the literature, according to MAFF scientists, so far as selenium content is concerned. No official explanation of this has been given, but it would seem likely that heat processing and modern agribusiness techniques profoundly reduce the selenium content of basic grain products.

Meat as a source of selenium looks good on most lists, and provides the major practical selenium source for the British way of life – liver and kidney being particularly rich sources. However, the selenium values for carcase meat, offal (and,

— FOOD SOURCES —

A short list of US values
(An up-to-date UK list does not exist, and generally speaking, transatlantic food is richer in selenium than *European food.*)

Selenium in µg per 100g edible portion (100g = 3½ oz)

Butter	146	Barley	24
Smoked herring	141	Eggs	21
Smelt	123	Orange juice	19
Wheatgerm	111	Gelatin	19
Brazil nuts	103	Beer	19
Apple cider vinegar	89	Beef liver and kidney	18
Scallops	77	Lamb chop	18
Wholewheat bread	66	Egg yolk	18
Lobster	65	Mushrooms	12
Bran	63	Chicken	12
Shrimps and prawns	59	Swiss cheese	10
Red Swiss chard	57	Cottage cheese	5
Oatflakes and meal	56	Wine	5
Clams, mussels	55	Radishes	4
Crab	51	Grape juice	4
Oysters	49	Pecan nuts	3
Milk	48	Hazelnuts	2
Cod	43	Almonds	2
Brown rice	34	Kidney beans	2
Lamb kidney	30	Onions	2
Turnips	27	Carrots	2
Garlic	25	Cabbage	2

Note: See main text for general comments on food sources.

incidentally, fish) are lower today than previously, and modern farming economy is probably implicated.

All in all it would seem that unless nuts, meat and offal are eaten in quantity and regularly, and cereal from North American sources is freely available and taken in substantial quantities, 'eating for selenium' is something of a lost cause in the 1990s. If we want to be sure we get enough selenium to enjoy its potential health benefits, then dietary supplementation seems to be the only practical way in the UK.

Do You Need Supplementation?

Regular, preferably daily, dietary supplementation is the most practical way of gaining health insurance from selenium. This is particularly so for those who have problems that hamper the absorption of trace elements. Within this probably substantial group are the elderly, the very young, those who self-select special diets (particularly low-calorie slimming diets), Vegans and the enormous group of 'idiopathic' poor absorbers. These are the aged, the impecunious pensioners whom we can only detect through the symptomatology of their chronic selenium depletion syndromes, and will probably be rheumatic sufferers, those with chronic arterial disease or certain cancer victims.

Recent reports from the Department of Health have now concluded that the RNI of selenium ($60-75\mu g$) seems on the low side. On the question of how long selenium supplements should be taken to maintain optimum health, little is known, unfortunately, about selenium storage in the body and the various factors that tend to antagonise selenium absorption. Unfortunately, too, tests for body content of selenium are both expensive and generally unobtainable, so the most sensible way to look at selenium dosage is to treat it like any other vital nutrient and take it daily in an amount that provides a degree of constant protection against selenium lack. Around $100\mu g$ per day seems adequate and carries no risk of overdosage.

ACNE AND SELENIUM

There are health foods better tailored for the skin disease acne – zinc, for instance – but selenium is useful too. Although not properly understood, the combination of selenium and Vitamin E can help clear up and prevent acne.

AGEING AND SELENIUM

It is the antioxidant action of selenium that can help slow down the ageing process, and many of the diseases that come with age.

Studies of the communities that are most long-lived – see page 165 – have shown that, apart from a good diet, the soil on which these peoples grow their food is selenium-rich.

ARTERY AND CARDIAC PROBLEMS AND SELENIUM

The arteries are particularly vulnerable to the ravages of the free radicals (see Glossary), and in at least two quite large studies it has been discovered that low levels of selenium in the blood are correlated to an increased risk of artery disease, manifesting itself in the form of stroke illness or coronary disease.

ARTHRITIS AND RHEUMATISM AND SELENIUM

Quite early in the history of selenium as a health food – in 1982 – the health magazine *Here's Health* published a trial that involved 100 people, all members of the Arthritic Association, who had severe and disabling arthritis. This group took Selenium-ACE (selenium, plus Vitamins A, C and E) and, although the trial was a small one and not blinded, the results were highly encouraging, for 70 per cent of the patients involved reported 'considerable improvement'.

To medical eyes Selenium-ACE initially appeared to be an unlikely formulation for a rheumatism remedy. But more recently a reappraisal has taken place, and selenium and the vitamins in question have now been acknowledged to be powerful antioxidants (see Glossary) and Free-radical quenchers.

CANCER AND SELENIUM

No causal link between selenium lack and the risk of a wide variety of cancers has been proved. But the possible dietary link between selenium and cancer persuades many people to take a daily dose of a selenium supplement as a prophylactic. This practice is supported by a careful study reported in the most prestigious US medical journal, the *New England Journal of Medicine*. This study involved the taking of samples of serum randomly from the population and storing them for five years, during which these population groups were carefully monitored to see if they developed cancer or not. The overall cancer risk for those with the selenium levels in the lowest of five levels was twice that of people with selenium levels in the highest level. Put more simply, people with *low* blood selenium are more likely to become cancer victims.

Another study of selenium and antioxidant cancer prevention was published recently in *GUT*, the world-famous gastroenterology journal, and earned selenium a tentative Gold Standard status in cancer prevention (tentative only, because the trial was a comparatively small one). Polyps in the large bowel are a well-recognised precursor to bowel cancer. Patients given selenium in a 200µg dosage for a month showed a significantly relevant reduction in the proliferating pre-cancer cells. Another similar study has been reported in the *European Journal of Cancer Prevention*.

A dietary study by Dr Roland Phillips, presented at a special symposium held on cancer and nutrition, compared the life and death statistics of two religious groups, the Seventh Day Adventists and the Mormons. Both follow a similar lifestyle in many ways, prohibiting alcohol and smoking, for instance, but Seventh Day Adventists are, generally speaking, vegetarians, as opposed to the meat-eating Mormons. The research revealed a possible link between meat-eating and cancer, for the Seventh Day Adventists developed cancer less frequently than did the Mormons.

But Dr Phillips did not stop there. He also showed that among the Mormons there were interesting variations in the cancer rate geographically. One group of theoretically cancer-prone, meat-eating Mormons had, in fact, a very low cancer rate. These were the Mormons who lived around Utah, and medical geography has discovered that this Utah area has a very high level of selenium in the soil. This, it would be reasonable to assume, was acting as a cancer preventative.

IMMUNODEPRESSION AND SELENIUM

A Brussels experiment involved 22 elderly residents of a nursing home in Brussels aged over 65, who had been institutionalised for over a year. Subjects were assigned to a six-month trial which involved the taking of either a selenium-enriched yeast in a 100µg daily dose or a placebo – the trial being of a double blind design. At the beginning of the trial the subjects' immune status was found to be lower than that of healthy adults. As the trial proceeded, however, this immunological response increased significantly, and eventually reached the upper normal limit for adults after six months' treatment.

This trial seems to be the first confirmation that a selenium-enriched yeast product can be immunostimulatory in elderly people. There was no remit as far as this trial was concerned to demonstrate that selenium has any prophylactic effect as far as colds or other illnesses are concerned. We must hope, however, that it will encourage others to pursue such work.

GOOD BUYS

There are many forms of selenium, but organic (yeast-based) selenium products have been proven to be 20 times more effective in building up blood selenium levels than inorganic selenium.

Selenium-ACE (WASSEN)
An excellent yeast-based organic product which is backed by extensive research and has a proven nutritional track record. It is a one-a-day supplement and contains 100µg of selenium plus Vitamins A, C and E to aid utilisation and absorption.

Selenium Bonus (LIFEPLAN)
An organic yeast-free formula containing 100µg of selenium for those who are allergic to yeast. It also contains other nutrients including beta-carotene, B vitamins, Vitamins C and E, zinc and chromium.

See also: **Glossary; Vitamins A, C, E; Acne; Ageing; Artery Problems; Arthritis and Rheumatism; Cancer; Cardiac Problems; Immunodepression.**

SULPHUR

ALTHOUGH by no means, strictly speaking, a *micro*nutrient, sulphur enters the body in small quantities in amino acids that are part and parcel of normal foodstuffs. Eggs, milk, meat and cereals all contain over 1 per cent of sulphur.

Sulphur sold as sulphate tablets is absorbed with difficulty and is largely excreted unchanged, and so is an extremely useless type of health food that is best left on the shelf.

VITAMIN A AND BETA-CAROTENE

VITAMIN A comes to us from Nature in two forms, as ß or beta-carotene or as Vitamin A 'proper'. Sometimes people wonder which is best, the plant-derived beta-carotene that our body converts into Vitamin A, or the actual animal-derived Vitamin A (or retinol). Nutritional science is still debating this point.

Although this vitamin has very definite and important health potential, it is also a vitamin to be watched carefully by the vitamin pill enthusiast, as in affluent societies overdosage probably causes more ill health than good. Those taking several supplements can be ingesting unsafe total dosages as far as Vitamin A is concerned, and over 500 cases of Vitamin A intoxication have been reported in over 200 separate reports, some of which included a fatal outcome. Sometimes confusion arises in as much as health-food shoppers are not all aware that beta-carotene is a *pro-vitamin* to Vitamin A and so contributes within the body to the total Vitamin A intake. It seems highly likely that beta-carotene will gain favour in health-food and medical circles because, being *water*-soluble, the kidneys excrete accidental or therapeutic excesses rather than the body storing it in the liver.

One of the reasons for doctors taking a rather casual attitude to Vitamin A deficiency these days is that many of us in an affluent society have very good stores of Vitamin A in our livers to fall back on, and so deficiency develops very slowly. Nevertheless, Vitamin A is required for the formation and maintenance of the epithelium (the mucous membranes of the body, including the eyes) and for the skin.

Signs and Symptoms of Deficiency

The best-understood symptom of Vitamin A deficiency is the development of night blindness and, indeed, the measurement of vision under adverse lighting forms a practical test for

Vitamin A deficiency. During the Second World War the Government exhorted the population to eat more carrots (rich in beta-carotene) to improve the necessary night vision to get around safely in blackout conditions and, indeed, a close watch was made on the night vision of RAF and other aircrew personnel for this reason. In affluent societies, gall bladder disease and malabsorption problems, which interfere with vitamin absorption, can sometimes be associated with night blindness.

Vitamin A also plays a vital part in the nutrition of the eye, particularly the colourless cornea and the conjunctiva that covers the eyeball. Severe and prolonged deprivation of adequate Vitamin A is responsible for upwards of half a million cases of blindness in children in the Third World.

Do You Need Supplementation?

In our society, only if you are a long-term faddy eater or dieter. In other words, people who don't like and won't eat liver, fish liver oils, dairy produce, eggs or fortified margarine, carrots, dark green leafy vegetables, apricots and melons are at risk of gradually exhausting their Vitamin A stores.

Strangely perhaps, not everyone is as well topped up with Vitamin A as some nutritional experts would argue. Several surveys of reasonably affluent groups in London and Canada (university students) were found to have very low stores of Vitamin A, and a post-mortem study of people (who had not died of Vitamin A deficiency) showed that 10 per cent had no measurable store of the vitamin in their livers at all. This seems to fly in the face of establishment nutritional assertions that we all have masses of the vitamin stored away in our bodies and so can virtually forget about it in our diet.

The most exciting facet of vitamin nutrition is a wealth of evidence that Vitamin A, and its pro-vitamin, beta-carotene, may play a part in protecting against a wide range of cancers, probably through an antioxidant action (see Glossary). Vitamin A also has valuable protective effects all over the body. A lack brings with it an increased liability to infection of the skin, respiratory system and of the urinogenital tract. It is important to stress that Vitamin A is protective and not curative in this type of action.

BALDING, SCALP AND HAIR PROBLEMS AND VITAMIN A

Some hair loss can be caused by a Vitamin A deficiency. Supplementation can help.

CANCER AND VITAMIN A

Several scientific papers (see Cancer) have reported that there is an association between low beta-carotene levels in blood, and cancers of the lung and larynx.

CATARACT AND VITAMIN A

Beta-carotene supplementation, investigated by several scientific sources (see Cataract), has proved effective in the prevention of cataract.

FIBROCYSTIC BREAST DISEASE AND VITAMIN A

Some studies have reported that Vitamin A can help, but the trials were small.

IMMUNODEPRESSION AND VITAMIN A

Immunological studies have shown that the more T-lymphocytes there are in the blood, the more the immune response is enhanced. Beta-carotene supplementation can bring this about.

ULCERATIVE COLITIS AND VITAMIN A

The oil-soluble Vitamins A and D, together with calcium, magnesium and zinc, have been reported to be useful in the management of ulcerative colitis (see also Crohn's Disease).

Dosages and Toxicity

Regular total intakes should not exceed 7,500µg per day for

women and 9,000 µg per day for men. Pregnant women should never exceed 3,300µg per day. For the purposes of checking total intakes, 6µg of beta-carotene is equivalent to 1µg of Vitamin A. Most health authorities recommend increasing the amount of beta-carotene in the total food intake. A meaningful amount to look for in a dietary supplement would be 400–450µg per day. In pregnancy, it should only be taken on medical recommendation.

Overdoses of Vitamin A can cause liver and bone damage, hair loss, double vision, headaches and birth defects.

Dietary Reference Values for Vitamin A, µg retinol equivalent

Age	LRNI		EAR		RNI	
	Males	Females	Males	Females	Males	Females
15–50+ yr	300	250	500	400	700	600

Additional amounts to be added to pre-pregnancy DRVs

Pregnant women	+ 100
Lactating women	+ 350

— FOOD SOURCES —

Beta-carotene
carrots; dark green leaf vegetables (spinach, broccoli); apricots; melon; pumpkin.

Vitamin A (retinol)
liver; fish liver oils; kidney; dairy produce; eggs; eel; fortified margarine.

In Britain about 35 per cent of needs comes from liver, 5 per cent from vegetables, and 5 per cent from milk and its products.

Vitamin A is very stable, an oil-soluble vitamin which resists almost all cooking processes, as well as storing remarkably well. The body stores it readily in the liver.

GOOD BUYS

Vitamin A is sold in two main forms, that of retinol derived from animal sources, and beta-carotene, or pro-vitamin A, which is derived from vegetable sources. One form of Vitamin A which is fairly inexpensive and has a very wide range of beneficial effects is cod liver oil (see page 25). Listed below are some more good quality and inexpensive forms of Vitamin A. Beta-carotene products are possibly a better buy than animal-source products.

Vitamin A (HEALTHCRAFTS)
Super Vitamin A (7,500 iu) capsules, and Natural Beta-carotene (15mg) capsules.

Vitamin A and Beta-carotene (HEALTHILIFE)
Vitamin A (2,500 iu) capsules and Beta-carotene (2,500 iu) capsules.

Beta-carotene (15mg) (QUEST)

See also: **Cod Liver Oil; Marine Oils; Balding and Scalp Hair Problems; Cancer; Cataract; Crohn's Disease; Fibrocystic Breast Disease; Immunodepression.**

VITAMIN B₁ (THIAMIN)

THE B VITAMIN complex is needed primarily for the enzyme system of digestion. Vitamin B_1 is particularly valuable in the metabolism or release of energy from carbohydrate foods – the more eaten, the more B_1 is required.

Unlike Vitamin A, Vitamin B_1 is so very soluble in water that 25 – 50 per cent of it boils out when we cook vegetables and fruit. We can minimise this. In the case of potatoes, a good practical source, boiling them in their skins destroys only 10 per cent of the vitamin. High-temperature cooking (roasting, frying) also destroys it. Baking powder has the same effect, so there is a reasonable case to be made for looking at Vitamin B_1 as a delicate nutrient, the benefits of which are incredibly easily lost to us. (For instance, pork is quite rich in B_1, but take your pork as pork sausages, and the meat preservative and the cooking rapidly destroy it.)

Signs and Symptoms of Deficiency

Beri-beri, the best-known B_1 deficiency disease, is now rare in the countries in which it was first described (Japan, Indonesia and Malaysia), but is still seen in chronic alcoholics the world over. Symptoms start with fatigue, feelings of numbness and stiffness of the legs which proceed to an inability to walk very far. Then come headaches, loss of appetite, loss of intellectual facility, and progressive paralysis. Sometimes patients on long-term bland diets for peptic ulcers develop similar symptoms. Beri-beri-type symptoms always develop very slowly as the body's stores are gradually exhausted. Those who eat normally, and include bread or flour products in reasonable amounts, are unlikely to need health-food supplements of Vitamin B_1.

Do You Need Supplementation?

It is difficult to see any protective effect operating as a result of the Vitamin B_1 that appears in multi-vitamin preparations, other than protecting the chronic alcoholic, the vagrant and those who put themselves on starvation or bizarre diets for long periods. But Vitamin B_1 helps a quicker recovery from gastrointestinal upsets and is given routinely to dialysis patients.

— FOOD SOURCES —

Whole germs of grains; whole-grain cereals, pasta, rice, flour; yeast; kidney, liver, pork.

Stability Factor
Cooking losses of the vitamin have already been mentioned. Chopping, mincing and liquidising reduce the Vitamin B_1 content by up to 75 per cent. Toasting bread (a major source) reduces the Vitamin B_1 content by up to 30 per cent, and canning of meat and vegetables can result in a loss of 30 per cent.

ALCOHOLISM AND VITAMIN B_1

A variation of beri-beri goes under an impressive name, the Wernicke-Korsakoff syndrome, which affects the eye muscles as well as the leg muscles, and is characterised by confusion, apathy, decreased awareness and amnesia. Unless intensively treated by Vitamin B_1, stupor, coma and permanent mental impairment occur. It occurs in alcoholics, those who starve themselves for various reasons, and is most likely to be seen in vagrants and those who have lost even their institutional homes and who live rough in the community.

HYPERKINESIS AND VITAMIN B_1

Some encouraging trials have been published relative to Vitamin B_1.

Dosage, Interactions and Toxicity

Department of Health Dietary Reference Values relate thiamin requirements to the number of calories taken daily. This involves complicated calculations that are unnecessary from the practical point of view, so I have reverted to the National Research Council's RDAs (Recommended Dietary Allowances 1989) which state that 1.0mg per day is the minimum recommended (plus 0.5mg per day in pregnancy).

Thiamin is easily excreted through the kidneys when taken in large amounts and doses of 500mg have been found to be non toxic even if taken for a month. Long-term mega intakes of more than 3g per day (about 1,000 times the RNI) may have undesirable effects in adults (headaches, irritability, insomnia, weakness, skin problems, rapid pulse).

Interactions occur with Levodopa, a drug used in the treatment of Parkinson's Disease. Levodopa should not be taken with Vitamin B_1.

See page 132 for recommended B_1 products.

See also: **Alcoholism; Hyperkinesis.**

VITAMIN B$_2$ (RIBOFLAVIN)

THE VITAMIN B$_2$ complex includes several substances, but riboflavin is particularly important. It helps in the way your body uses carbohydrates and proteins, and is required for the production of antibodies. It is linked to the absorption of iron, as well as Vitamin B$_6$ and folate, or folic acid.

There are no stores of riboflavin in the body, but the vitamin is present widely in almost all foods, and so supplemental B$_2$ is seldom necessary in the ordinary way of life. The body also regularly excretes Vitamin B$_2$ in healthy eaters, indicating that most of us take in more than we need. This is odd, perhaps, because Vitamin B$_2$ is so very insoluble, and this limits absorption to such an extent that even massive intakes of the vitamin do not seem to do us any harm! Veterinary medicine tells us that Vitamin B$_2$ is important for the healthy raising of a variety of domestic animals, and so it should come as no great surprise that we need it too. But exactly why some people need Vitamin B$_2$ as a health food supplement to them away from deficiency problems remains a mystery.

Signs and Symptoms of Deficiency

The 'ifs' and 'buts' that characterise Vitamin B$_2$ bedevil its symptomatology. It is quite easy to pinpoint one of the main symptoms of Vitamin B$_2$ deficiency (a tendency to sores and splits in the skin around the corners of the mouth), but this sympton is often quite unrelated to B$_2$ intake. A sore, red tongue occurs in B$_2$ deficiency, as it does in anaemia and Vitamin C deficiency. A scaly sort of eczematous dermatitis around the face, especially the sides of the nose, commonly but not exclusively occurs in Vitamin B$_2$ deficiency.

Do You Need Supplementation?

Those who drink no milk and/or eat no cheese are ignoring prime dietary sources of B$_2$. Pregnant women suffering from

119

thyrotoxicosis (over production of thryoid hormone, also called hyperthyroidism), patients taking Chlorpromazine, Impiramine or Amitriptyline, and patients on dialysis need extra Vitamin B$_2$ too.

— FOOD SOURCES —

Liver, kidney; milk, yoghurt; cheese; Marmite; eggs; wheatgerm; wheat bran; mushrooms; fortified cereals.

In Britain, on average, milk and cheese supply about 40 per cent of needs.

Vitamin B$_{95}$ is relatively stable but is adversely affected by exposure to sunlight. Milk left on doorsteps loses some of its B$_2$ content as the day passes.

Dosage

It is unlikely that high intakes are dangerous due to Vitamin B$_2$'s poor solubility, and this makes minimum dosage the principal interest. RNIs of 1mg per day are adequate for children and adults.

Doctors often prescribe Vitamin B$_2$ in 10mg doses (or in a multiple B complex tablet). It would seem that Vitamin B$_2$ is a suitable health-food supplement even if we don't quite understand why.

See page 132 for recommended B$_2$ products.

VITAMIN B₃ (NIACIN)

INTEREST in this vitamin – known as both niacin and nicotinic acid – centres on the fact that if you live off a diet of maize and virtually nothing else you develop a disease called pellagra. This is characterised, as every medical student will tell you, by the three Ds, dermatitis, diarrhoea and dementia. It used to be prevalent in India, Asia and the Southern USA, but is now rare except in Bantu Africa and in very primitive parts of India. It can occur in this country, as testified by Hugh Sinclair, the eminent nutritionist, in his and D.F. Hollingsworth's classic book *Hutchison's Food and the Principles of Nutrition*, in demented patients in mental hospitals; in them the dementia may be the presenting symptom of pellagra (rather than the other two Ds).

The present clinical fashion for relocating mentally disturbed people in the community rather than in institutions brings with it the long shadow of Vitamin B₃ deficiency. Because such patients are notoriously difficult to feed properly, it is worthwhile considering the necessity of regular Vitamin B₃ supplementation.

The fact that brewer's yeast is rich in Vitamin B₃ probably explains the erstwhile popularity of that product as a health food.

Large doses of Vitamin B₃ have been used to lower blood cholesterol and lipids. This cardiovascular nutrient therapy provides an interesting bridge between the world of health-food manipulation and general medicine.

Signs and Symptoms of Deficiency

These have already been noted, but the classical D triad may not always be present in its entirety. Sores and ulcers in the mouth can be a symptom as well.

Do You Need Supplementation?

In all probability only those do who for one reason or another starve themselves or live on bizarre diets for long periods.

— FOOD SOURCES —

Liver, kidney; meat; fish; brewer's yeast; Marmite; peanuts; bran; pulses; wholemeal wheat; coffee.

In Britain, on average, meats and meat products supply about 35 per cent of needs.

Vitamin B_3 is incredibly stable and resists even the most traumatic culinary and storage processes.

DYSMENORRHOEA AND VITAMIN B_3

In a study in the 1950s (see page 224), women who suffered from dysmenorrhoea were given niacin before and during menstruation. It helped in 90 per cent of cases. Nothing much seems to have been done since in the way of effective trials, but niacin still can be of considerable benefit.

HYPERKINESIS AND VITAMIN B_3

Some encouraging results have been shown by B complex supplementation.

POOR CIRCULATION (CHILBLAINS) AND VITAMIN B_3

Because Vitamin B_3 in large doses causes skin flushing, this galvanises the circulation, and it has gained a well-earned reputation for the treatment of chilblains. Large doses, 100mg and above, are prescribed.

Dosage and Contraindications

The table below gives information that relates to dietary units of 1,000 kcal per day. Those who do not wish to enter into this nutritional sophistication can rest assured that 10 – 15mg per day is a reasonable dosage, should they find themselves dealing with a person who refuses to eat on a long-term basis, and can be assumed to be a meaningful amount in the vitamin supplement.

Dietary Reference Values for Niacin – mg niacin equivalent/1,000 kcal food intake per day

Age	LRNI	EAR	RNI
All ages	4.4	5.5	6.6

Additional amounts to be added to pre-pregnancy DRVs

Lactating women	+ 2.3mg per day

Peptic ulcer sufferers should not take Vitamin B₃ products.

See page 132 for recommended B₃ products.

See also: **Dysmenorrhoea; Hyperkinesis; Poor Circulation (Chilblains).**

VITAMIN B$_6$ (PYRIDOXINE)

THIS vitamin is not a single substance, but a complex of several related compounds, the best-known of which is pyridoxine. Vitamin B$_6$ has been misused in high doses for the management of PMS (pre-menstrual syndrome), and is somewhat out of fashion as a result, although some considerable evidence exists that it is valuable in the management of that curious and somewhat baffling condition when used in sensible doses.

Vitamin B$_6$ is required for amino acid metabolism.

Signs and Symptoms of Deficiency

These are rather difficult because *symptoms* of deficiency – PMS, food allergy, depression, for instance – usually erupt before *signs* – a form of dietary dermatitis, for instance – occur.

— FOOD SOURCES —

Liver, kidney; whole-grain cereals; meat; fish; peanuts; bananas; walnuts; avocados; potatoes; eggs; royal jelly.

Vitamin B$_6$ is relatively stable but losses can occur in cooking.

Do You Need Supplementation?

As a health food, probably no. To a large extent, those who are at risk of deficiency are special groups of patients undergoing medical treatments, for example those taking Hydralazine for hypertension, Penicillamine for arthritis, and oestrogens. Pharmacological rather than health-food doses are prescribed by doctors to treat certain rare kidney and blood problems. Very high doses (above 500mg per day) may produce symptoms of (reversible) neuritis (numbness of legs).

ACNE AND VITAMIN B$_6$

Small and safe doses of Vitamin B$_6$ may well help acne if it is the sort that seems to come and go with periods or with PMS. Large-scale corroborative evidence in the medical press is scanty, although in one study of 106 young women, over 75 per cent benefited as far as their acne was concerned by taking 50mg daily of B$_6$ (a safe dose) for a week prior to menstruation and during their period.

ALLERGY (FOOD) AND VITAMIN B$_6$

Dosages of 50mg per day for twelve weeks have cured many people's sensitivity to foods, particularly those containing MSG (monosodium glutamate).

CARPAL TUNNEL SYNDROME AND VITAMIN B$_6$

There has been some research into the effects of pyridoxine on patients, usually women, suffering from this hand problem. Surgery is usually the answer, but for those who fear the knife, a daily dose of up to 100mg (no more) could possibly be of benefit.

DEPRESSION AND VITAMIN B$_6$

The oestrogens contained in the contraceptive pill can bring about a form of depression. This has been improved, in a placebo-controlled study, by pyridoxine therapy.

DYSMENORRHOEA AND VITAMIN B$_6$

Pyridoxine and magnesium therapy has been shown to benefit the pain and cramps of dysmenorrhoea. This treatment would be suitable for those who look for a gentle and non-analgesic solution to the problem.

HYPERKINESIS AND VITAMIN B$_6$

Supplementation with B complex vitamins has shown some improvement in over-active children.

KIDNEY STONES AND VITAMIN B$_6$

There is some evidence that Vitamin B$_6$ can inhibit kidney stone formation, especially when taken in conjunction with magnesium.

PMS AND VITAMIN B$_6$

Both anxiety-dominated PMS and the 'bloating' variety – PMS-H – can be alleviated sometimes by Vitamin B$_6$, but the therapy is less valued now than it once was.

Dosage and Toxicity

Widely popular as a dietary supplement in the management of pre-menstrual tension, there have been several recent concerns with reference to possible toxicity when large doses of Vitamin B$_6$ are taken over a prolonged period. (The average dosage in B$_6$ toxicity involved taking over 100mg per day.) Toxic symptoms (neuropathy) usually disappear on cessation of dosage.

High intakes have been associated with a reversible impaired function of the sensory nerves in excess of an intake level of 50mg per day, and even this dosage should be viewed with caution. Further research will be necessary to confirm a totally safe dose. Over-enthusiastic vitamin pill poppers who mix their vitamins unwisely could put themselves at risk of developing overdosage symptoms, although in most cases *very* large doses are necessary to bring about the tingling or numbness associated with sensory nerve problems. Doses of 2–7g per day have caused nerve damage.

DRVs are based on a dietary intake of specific amounts of energy protein. More practical are more old-fashioned National Research Council assessments of 1.5 – 2mg daily.

See page 132 – 3 for recommended B$_6$ products.

See also: **Magnesium; Acne; Allergy; Carpal Tunnel Syndrome; Depression; Dysmenorrhoea; Hyperkinesis; Kidney Stones; PMS.**

VITAMIN B$_{12}$

VITAMIN B$_{12}$ is our youngest vitamin, and was not isolated until 1948 (from liver, and used for the treatment of pernicious anaemia). It is found only in animal foods, and so Vegans are at special risk of deficiency. There is an interesting nutritional link between Vitamin B$_{12}$ and folate, in as much as they are both vital to the synthesis of DNA, and the efficient workings of the nervous system. The whole story of Vitamin B$_{12}$ is one of quite exhilarating economy of intake and yet massive storage by the body: we eat about 5mg in our food each day, absorb about 1mg of this, yet store some 1,000mg in our liver! As we 'use' and excrete only very small quantities of B$_{12}$ each day, it takes a long time before anyone starts to get deficient, even on a Vitamin B$_{12}$-free (Vegan) diet.

B$_{12}$ is required by the bone marrow, for red blood cell formation and maturation, and the function of the whole central nervous system.

Signs and Symptoms of Deficiency

These include anaemia symptoms (breathlessness, some vague tiredness and pallor), weight loss and various mental and neurological symptoms. The reasons for the deficiency can be

1) dietary, 2) disease of the gastrointestinal tract causing malabsorption, 3) heavy worm infestation, or 4) congenital problems.

The major B$_{12}$ deficiency disease is pernicious anaemia, which develops not through a dietary lack, but through an inability to *absorb* the vitamin.

Do You Need Supplementation?

Yes, if you are a Vegan or a victim of any of the diseases causing malabsorption of nutrients generally: for example, pernicious anaemia, Crohn's Disease, some diabetics and MS victims, and those on long-term drug routines.

There is a conviction very prevalent among some people (mostly Asians) that they feel very much better as far as their general health is concerned if they receive regular injections of Vitamin B$_{12}$, even if blood tests pronounce them not deficient in the vitamin and they are taking an adequate diet. There is no method of measuring or exploring the satisfaction experienced through even prolonged medication with Vitamin B$_{12}$ so, in the face of medical scepticism, the practice continues. Oral Vitamin B$_{12}$ is included in many multi-vitamin preparations.

— FOOD SOURCES —

Liver, kidney; sardines; oysters; meats; eggs; cheese; milk.

It is extremely stable, and resists storage, freezing and canning for several years.

Dosage

High intakes are not dangerous, so minimum intakes for all ages can be generous, and RNIs of around 1.5µg per day are reasonable.

See page 133 for recommended B$_{12}$ products.

FOLATE (FOLIC ACID)

THE words folate and folic come from the Latin for leaf, and many green leafy foods contain significant amounts of this B complex vitamin. Folate works with B_{12} and C in the metabolism of proteins, and is important for the division of cells.

In contrast to Vitamin B_{12}, we store only a very little folate in our bodies, and so in the cases of poor intake or malabsorption, or drugs interfering with absorption, folate deficiencies can develop quite rapidly. If this occurs at the moment of conception there is a higher than average risk of spina bifida or other malformation in any foetus conceived at that time. However, a good diet will ensure good folate levels in the body.

Signs and Symptoms of Deficiency

If this book had been written before the 1990s it would have dismissed folate deficiency by mentioning a fairly rare type of anaemia, occurring in the tropics or sometimes in pregnancy. The symptoms of this quite rare problem include a sore tongue and minor gastrointestinal disturbances. A mention might have been made that *some* nutritionists believed that folate deficiency in pregnancy was associated with a tragic form of abnormality in new-born babies, neural-tube defect or spina bifida, but that the subject was still being debated. Then in early 1991 the *Lancet* published the results of the Medical Research Council's Vitamin Study Group which confirmed that folic acid supplementation has a very high (72 per cent) protective effect as far as spina bifida is concerned, even in high-risk-group women (those who have been previously delivered of a neural-tube defective baby).

As a result the nutritional powers that be now recommend that all women *at risk of pregnancy* should take adequate amounts of folate in their diet, or folate supplements. Nobody as yet knows *why* so many women need prophylactic folate at the time of conception. It could be an absorption problem, but it could also be an environmental problem, as yet unidentified.

Do You Need Supplementation?

Yes, is the short and snappy answer, if there is any chance of your becoming pregnant.

Forward-looking health authorities are already issuing folate to women trying to conceive, in the form of Pregnavite Forte F which contains 0.36mg of folate. When the emotional effects of experiencing neural-tube defect in the family are considered, together with the financial and other burdens that the disease places on health services in the community, it is incredible that *all* women planning a pregnancy are not advised to take supplementary folate.

Many drugs, in particular alcohol and antibiotics, can bring about folate malabsorption.

It is important that folate should not be self-selected as a 'blood tonic' for although it remits the anaemia of per-nicious anaemia, it does not prevent the development of neurological complications of that disease (Vitamin B_{12} can help both).

— FOOD SOURCES —

Wheatgerm; yeast extract; liver; kidney; spinach; broccoli; some beans; beetroot; bran; raw peanuts; cabbage; lettuce; avocados; bananas; oranges; wholemeal bread; eggs; some fish.

In Britain vegetables provide 35 per cent, bread and flour products 26 per cent, fruit 6 per cent of needs.

Folate is a relatively stable compound unless it is cooked with high nitrate-concentration water. How important this is requires further exploration.

CERVICAL CANCER AND FOLATE

A few years ago an article in a US obstetrics and gynae-cology journal demonstrated that blood levels of folate are lower in cervical cancer patients than in control subjects. A previous study had also shown that so-called cervical dysplasia (an abnormality sometimes noted on routine cervical smear tests that can progress to cervical cancer if untreated) could be improved if such patients are treated by folate supplementation. This seems to be a nutritional link between health-food therapy and cancer that is difficult to ignore.

Dosages and Interactions

Interactions can lead to reduced zinc absorption.

Dietary Reference Values for Folate, µg per day

Age	LRNI	EAR	RNI
11 + yr	100	150	200
Additional amounts to be added to pre-pregnancy DRVs			
Pregnant women	+ 100		
Lactating women	+ 60		

See page 133 for recommended folate products.

See also: **Birth Defects; Cancer.**

GOOD BUYS – VITAMIN B COMPLEX

There is very little to choose between the products of manufacturers as far as these vitamins are concerned, most of which are marketed in 'multi' forms. Sustained-release products have little to recommend them over other preparations. Availability and relative price will sensibly dictate choice.

VITAMIN B$_1$

Vitamin B$_1$, or thiamin, is available in a variety of strengths. It is not such a common product as many of the other vitamins, but if it is not available at your local health-food store it can be obtained by mail order.

Vitamin B$_1$ (100mg) (BLACKMORE'S)

Vitamin B$_1$ (100mg) (CANTASSIUM)

VITAMIN B$_2$

Vitamin B$_2$ or riboflavin is another vitamin which is not common in all health food shops. It can be ordered by mail in case of difficulty.

Vitamin B$_2$ (50mg) (BLACKMORE'S)

Vitamin B$_2$ (25mg) (CANTASSIUM)

VITAMIN B$_3$

Vitamin B$_3$ is also known as nicotinic acid, niacin or nicotinamide.

Vitamin B$_3$ (250mg) (BLACKMORE'S)

Vitamin B$_3$ Nicotinamide (100/500mg) (CANTASSIUM)

Vitamin B$_3$ Niacin (100mg) (NATURAL FLOW)

VITAMIN B$_6$

Vitamin B$_6$ is also known as pyridoxine.

Vitamin B$_6$ (100mg) (BLACKMORE'S)

Vitamin B$_6$ (50mg) (CANTASSIUM)

VITAMIN B$_{12}$

Vitamin B$_{12}$ (100μg) BLACKMORE'S)

Vitamin B$_{12}$ (50μg) (CANTASSIUM)

FOLATE

Folate is also known as folic acid.

Folic Acid (100/500μg) (CANTASSIUM)

Folic Acid (800μg) (NATURAL FLOW)
Folic acid is also available in NHS multi-vitamin products. Pregnavite Forte F (Bencard) is the best-established of these.

BIOTIN

This is a B-group vitamin of which very little is needed in the diet (it is present in most foods, particularly kidney and yeast). The only deficiency known is that caused by massive over-consumption of egg white (which contains an antivitamin).

VITAMIN C

IT was a naval surgeon called Lind who did the first controlled nutrition trial on his shipmates on HMS *Salisbury* in 1747: he showed that citrus fruit and juice cured scurvy – a disease that decimated sailors on long ocean voyages at the time. Vitamin C is an interesting substance in that humans, other primates and guinea pigs are different from the rest of the animal world: they cannot manufacture their own Vitamin C, and so have to rely on dietary sources.

For some years there have been advocates of megadoses (up to 10g per day) of Vitamin C producing a sort of 'superhealth'. The fact that a prominent advocate in this field was a Nobel Laureate, Linus Pauling, gave credence to the practice and launched nutritionists on an unusually enthusiastic number of clinical trials. One of the contentions of the megavitamin lobby was that the practice prevented colds. An analysis of the results of 31 controlled trials showed no significant protective effect in 23 of them, and in the supportive trials cynical scientific appraisal pointed out that they were not double blind, had small numbers, or showed benefit only in subgroups. Megatherapy is also beset with disadvantages, producing diarrhoea, dyspepsia and an increased incidence of kidney stones. Many takers also sometimes had subsequent difficulty in absorbing enough of the vitamin when they reverted to normal intakes, and so developed mild scurvy unless they took extra Vitamin C for life!

A more modern health bonus exists in that Vitamin C is an antioxidant, along with Vitamins A and E, and the micronutrient selenium (see Glossary). These substances are gaining an enviable reputation with reference to playing a part in the protection of the body from oxidant damage, which includes at least some cancers and arteriosclerotic disease.

Signs and Symptoms of Deficiency

Scurvy as such only occurs quite rarely these days, although it has become recognised that a pre-scurvy syndrome – characterised by weakness, aches and pains – exists in those who do not get enough Vitamin C-rich foodstuffs. A blood test can confirm the deficiency, and treatment with large doses of the vitamin soon cures the condition. Other symptoms suggestive of Vitamin C deficiency include a curious 'cork-screw' deformity of the hair, spongy, bleeding gums (one of the signs of scurvy), spontaneous bruising, anaemia and failures of wound healing. The last-named occurs because of Vitamin C's role in the manufacture of collagen, a substance which forms the connective tissues in skin; if C is deficient in the diet, tissues can be less effective in action, and any wounds heal more slowly and less efficiently.

Do You Need Supplementation?

All infants are at special risk unless they are given supplementary Vitamin C as orange juice. Breast-fed infants get adequate amounts of Vitamin C, but only if their mother's intake is adequate. Patients in hospital, people in institutions or old people's homes will rarely get enough Vitamin C due to the very nature of even the best institutional cooking. Whether or not they need supplements depends on the frequency of fresh fruit and salads on the menu. Those who have recently had operations will need supplements of Vitamin C to promote healthy wound healing. The present fashion for day-care surgery means that home convalescence often needs to look at adequate post-operative Vitamin C intake.

ANAEMIA AND VITAMIN C

Iron is the Gold Standard health food in the treatment of dietary anaemia, and Vitamin C helps in its absorption. Many health food products combine the two for this reason.

— FOOD SOURCES —

Blackcurrants; guavas; rosehip syrup; green peppers; oranges and other fruits; vegetaables of the brassica family (cauliflower, broccoli, Brussels sprouts, cabbage); sprouted pulses; potatoes; liver and milk.

In Britain on average vegetables supply about 48 per cent of needs (about 20 per cent from potatoes); fruits contribute about 40 per cent.

Vitamin C is the most unstable and easily destroyed of the vitamins – so much so that to estimate the Vitamin C content of any foodstuff at any time is little better than a guesstimate. Up to 50 per cent of the vitamin is destroyed by even rapid cooking. Oxygen is also a major culprit as far as Vitamin C destruction is concerned: for instance, cutting up a vegetable well in advance of cooking means that most of its C content is lost. Peeling, handling, washing can all cause loss of Vitamin C.

The effect of storage on fruit juice is interesting. It retains its vitamin content quite well until it is opened (due to sulphur dioxide preservative content), but it loses half its Vitamin C within 8 days of initial opening.

Because relatively little Vitamin C may be stored, daily vitamin supplements rather than food are the safest ways of being sure of a constant adequate intake, especially during the winter months.

ARTERY PROBLEMS AND VITAMIN C

It is Vitamin C's antioxidant properties that are significant here. There is some evidence that a marginal but persistent Vitamin C deficiency may contribute to the development of atherosclerosis (degenerative disease of the arteries). Several clinical trials using relatively large doses of Vitamin C (1g twice or three times daily) have been followed by changes in blood chemistry that suggest that Vitamin C supplementation is beneficial in preventing artery disease.

BALDING, SCALP AND HAIR PROBLEMS AND VITAMIN C

As mentioned, hair can become misshapen and tangled due to a severe Vitamin C deficiency. Scalp dryness and hair loss can be prevented by daily supplementation with C.

BED SORES AND VITAMIN C

Probably because of its wound-healing qualities, Vitamin C has proved very effective in the treatment of pressure sore ulceration.

CATARACT AND VITAMIN C

Dietary factors are being viewed as increasingly significant in the prevention of cataracts, and chief among the health-food aids are the antioxidant Vitamins A (in the form of beta-carotene), C and E.

GALL BLADDER PROBLEMS AND VITAMIN C

Research has suggested that extra Vitamin C (or E) can suppress gallstone formation.

HERPES AND VITAMIN C

Vitamin C supplementation has been proven in trials to decrease the duration of herpes attacks.

HYPERKINESIS AND VITAMIN C

Some trials have suggested that mega C doses are useful in hyperkinesis management.

LARYNX CANCER AND VITAMIN C

Both smoking and excess alcohol intake are associated with cancer of the voicebox, and it is well known that both these habits reduce the levels of Vitamin C in the body. Low levels of

Vitamin C (and of A) in the diet have been linked to the development of larynx cancer.

MENORRHAGIA AND VITAMIN C

Once more, because it assists the absorption of iron, Vitamin C can help the potential anaemia in young and healthy sufferers from menorrhagia, or heavy periods.

PERIODONTAL DISEASE AND VITAMIN C

The curative power of Vitamin C in relation to bleeding gums was proved very early on, in the treatment of scurvy. Its abilities can be used to good effect in the treatment and prevention of other periodontal problems.

TIREDNESS, FATIGUE AND VITAMIN C

When used to reinforce iron supplements, Vitamin C can help overcome the tiredness that is symptomatic of anaemia.

Dosage and Interactions

There are several drugs that antagonise Vitamin C, including steroids, aspirin, indomethacin, phenylbutazone and tetra-cyclines. Smoking and excess alcohol also inhibit Vitamin C's action. The elderly need to consider their Vitamin C status on a long-term basis, particularly if they lack teeth or have false teeth as they will be disinclined to eat many Vitamin C-rich foodstuffs.

Dietary Reference Values for Vitamin C, mg per day

Age	LRNI	EAR	RNI
15 + yr	10	25	40
Additional amounts to be added to pre-pregnancy DRVs			
Pregnant women		+ 10	
Lactating women		+ 30	

Many would agree that these Department of Health DRVs are too low. When selecting a daily dietary supplement for high-risk groups a dose in excess of 40mg per day would be advisable. Post-operatively, 250mg per day would be a reasonable intake.

GOOD BUYS

It is difficult to choose between available products due to their intrinsic similarity. You should shop sensibly with price and availability in mind.

Quest Range
This range of Vitamin C products caters for several needs. A chewable formula is useful for those who do not like swallowing tablets or who prefer a natural-tasting product. A complete C-plus complex with bioflavonoids, containing 500mg of Vitamin C and 500mg of bioflavonoids, is available, a timed-release formula, plus a low-acid buffered formula for those whose digestive systems have difficulty coping with acid substances like Vitamin C.

Healthcrafts Range
This is also a range which covers a variety of needs. It consists of a fruit-flavoured chewable Vitamin C, Super Vitamin C containing 500mg, High Potency Vitamin C containing 1g, PRN Mega-C 1500, a prolonged-release tablet giving 1,500mg, Vitamin C and E, a combination formula containing 500mg of Vitamin C and 400 iu of Vitamin E, and finally Vitamin C and zinc lozenges containing 300mg of Vitamin C and 7mg of zinc.

Blackmore's Range
This is a high-quality range of Vitamin C products which includes a 500mg formula with a vegetable protein coating.

See also: **Anaemia; Artery Problems; Balding, Scalp and Hair Problems; Bedsores; Cancer; Cataract; Gall Bladder Problems; Herpes; Hyperkinesis; Menorrhagia; Periodontal Disease; Tiredness and fatigue.**

VITAMIN D

VITAMIN D was of great interest in the past – once it became widely known that cod liver oil was a sure cure for rickets – but is now of less importance nutritionally, particularly because margarines are fortified with it. Vitamin D occurs in very few foods (see page 141), but the skin manufactures it in sunlight. Provided we spend a certain amount of time out of doors each day, especially in the summer, and expose the skin, then the body will have sufficient stores to keep us free of problems for most of the year.

In winter, the diet may have to be relied on. People with dark skins living in northern latitudes have a problem, as their skins were designed for a much fiercer sun, and therefore may not manufacture sufficient D.

Vitamin D is required for the absorption and use of calcium, and this is particularly important for babies and young children because calcium is vital for the formation and hardening of bones and teeth. Vitamin D also promotes the absorption of zinc by the body. However, D increases the body's requirements of magnesium: all the D-fortified foods (such as margarine and baby milks) could, particularly in the young, lead to a deficiency of magnesium.

Signs and Symptoms of Deficiency

Bone and muscle pain are early symptoms of rickets, but because victims are usually children between six months and three years these tend to go unheeded. Bone deformity – because the bones have calcified abnormally – finally discloses the full clinical picture of rickets. Badly-formed teeth in children can result from a deficiency of Vitamin D, probably because of the relationship between D and calcium.

Do You Need Supplementation?

Those who spend most of their time indoors and only venture

outside when heavily clothed – babies and elderly people in the main – are at risk of Vitamin D deficiency. Children who do not eat Vitamin D-rich foods and all coloured races living in northern latitudes are potentially in need of supplementation, especially towards the end of the winter, when summer stores of the vitamin are becoming depleted.

Vegans, who will not take fish or fish oils, are sometimes at risk, especially in the coloured races. Patients who are epileptic and take phenobarbitone or phenytoin may need supplementation, as these drugs inhibit Vitamin D synthesis.

— FOOD SOURCES —

Fish liver oils; fatty fish (sardines, herring, mackerel, tuna, salmon, pilchards); fortified margarine; infant milk formulae; eggs; liver.

In Britain, on average, margarine supplies around 54 per cent of needs.

Vitamin D is very stable.

OSTEOPOROSIS AND VITAMIN D

Vitamin D, together with the parathyroid gland, is responsible for regulating the balance between the calcium in the bones and the calcium concentration in the blood. A deficiency, therefore, can affect the mineralisation of the bones, which is highly interesting in the light of the most recent research (1992) hailing from Addenbrooke's Hospital, University of Cambridge. This suggests that if the present intake of Vitamin D is increased to 400 iu per day, it would result in a considerable increase in bone density.

A Vitamin D supplement is particularly useful for older males, who should make sure of that 400 iu daily.

ULCERATIVE COLITIS AND VITAMIN D

There is some evidence that the antioxidant vitamins A and D, together with calcium, magnesium and zinc, can play a useful therapeutic part in the management of the disease (see Crohn's Disease).

Dosage, Toxicity and Contraindications

Excessively high intakes of Vitamin D are more dangerous for infants than for adults. Intakes of 50μg per day have been associated with high blood calcium troubles; these can lead to hypercalcaemia, calcium deposits in the heart and kidneys. Problems can occur at only five times the RDA in sunny climes. Intake must never be more than 1,800 iu or 45μg per day.

Dietary Reference Values for Vitamin D, μg per day

Age	RNI
0 – up to 6 months	8.5
6 months – 3 yr	7.0
4 – 64 yr	0 provided that the skin is exposed to the sun reasonably often.
65 + yr	10.0
Pregnant and lactating women	10.0

Beware of hypervitaminosis through taking other vitamin preparations. Take special precautions, in the form of medical advice, in kidney disease, sarcoidosis (a disease characterized by lumps in the skin, thinning of finger bones and changes in the lung similar to tuberculosis), and pregnancy.

GOOD BUYS

Vitamin A + D (QUEST)

Marine Oil Products
Sanatogen Cod Liver Oil is excellent value for money.

Seven Seas Cod Liver Oil: the manufacturers have gone to considerable pains to combat the 'cod liver oil taste' in many of their products.

See also: **Calcium; Cod Liver Oil; Magnesium; Marine Oils; Zinc; Crohn's Disease; Osteoporosis; Rickets.**

VITAMIN E

FOR some years Vitamin E has been a substance that medical science could not make up its mind about. Like Vitamins A and D, it is an oily substance which occurs in vegetable oils and to some extent in fish. The part that it plays in human nutrition is still being debated.

There are several odd facts about Vitamin E that (just) dissuade cynical nutritionists from dismissing it as a less than therapeutically exciting health food product. For instance, it prevents a form of blindness in new-born babies that have been subjected to oxygen therapy. Then there are patients who for various reasons have severe problems over the absorption of fat and develop a form of anaemia and certain neurological problems which respond to Vitamin E therapy.

Probably Vitamin E's most important role is as a member of that élite corps of health foods known as antioxidants (see Glossary). As such, together with Vitamins A (beta-carotene), C and the micronutrient selenium, Vitamin E may well have health bonuses that at the present state of the nutritional art are not fully appreciated. As a fatty antioxidant it is particularly involved with the protection of polyunsaturates from oxidation to less healthy fats and oils in the body. The more poly-unsaturated fat (PUFA) there is in your diet (the more *healthy* fat, some would say), the more Vitamin E you need to cope with it in a complex biochemical way.

Signs and Symptoms of Deficiency

Vitamin E's previous somewhat questionable reputation has probably evolved more as a result of false claims for vitamin magic than most other vitamins. For instance, today most nutritionists agree that Vitamin E does *not* promote sexual prowess, athletic achievement, or play a major part in the management of ageing or infertility, as has been previously claimed. However, as a useful preventative antioxidant, it probably *is* a coronary and other artery protective.

Do You Need Supplementation?

Probably only those who have long-standing fat absorption problems and new-born children subjected to oxygen therapy have substantial needs, but as a very stable antioxidant it is clearly of great value.

— FOOD SOURCES —

Vegetable oils (wheatgerm oil is the richest); margarines; eggs; butter; wholemeal cereals; bread; broccoli.

Vitamin E differs from all other vitamins in that it is unstable when frozen. In this age of the deep-freeze, 8 weeks of freezing can produce an 80 per cent loss in the Vitamin E content of foods. Heat also adversely affects Vitamin E content, reducing it by about 30 per cent; bread-baking reduces the original grain Vitamin E content by 58 per cent. Perhaps in the face of Vitamin E's inherent instability, and despite its only partially accepted health bonuses, its inclusion in many multiple-vitamin health foods is not all that stupid.

ACNE AND VITAMIN E

Several companies produce Vitamin E creams which are said to prevent and reduce wrinkles in the skin. There is no proof at all that there is any real therapeutic value in this, but Vitamin E taken with the micronutrient selenium can help clear up and prevent acne.

ARTERY PROBLEMS AND VITAMIN E

There is some indication that the antioxidant Vitamins A (beta-carotene), C and E, plus selenium, can protect the arteries from damage.

CATARACT AND VITAMIN E

There is quite a considerable body of evidence that relates health of the eyes to the antioxidant vitamins.

DIABETES AND VITAMIN E

One study of diabetes suggested that diabetics who include Vitamin E in their diets might possibly need to reduce their requirement of insulin.

DYSMENORRHOEA AND VITAMIN E

A trial in the 1950s showed a considerable improvement in those receiving Vitamin E over those receiving the placebo.

FIBROCYSTIC BREAST DISEASE AND VITAMIN E

Some studies have reported that E can help, but the trials were small.

GALL BLADDER PROBLEMS AND VITAMIN E

Research has suggested that extra Vitamin E (or C) can suppress gallstone formation.

IMMUNODEPRESSION AND VITAMIN E

The antioxidant vitamins have been identified as beneficial to the immune system.

LARYNX CANCER AND VITAMIN E

There is some evidence that a shortage of Vitamins C and E can increase the risks of this cancer.

MENOPAUSAL PROBLEMS AND VITAMIN E

At least four trials have demonstrated that Vitamin E can benefit menopausal women.

MENORRHAGIA AND VITAMIN E

One study involving Vitamin E supplementation revealed diminished blood loss in the trial group of women suffering menorrhagia associated with IUD usage.

PMS AND VITAMIN E

The 'bloating' form of PMS – PMS-H – and breast tenderness in particular, can sometimes be alleviated by Vitamin E therapy.

Dosage

The most recent Department of Health review finds it impossible to set DRVs of practical value, but suggests that 3 to 4 mg of Vitamin E, in alpha tocopherol form, is adequate. Other authorities suggest an adequate intake is 10–15mg of the vitamin (as tocopherol acetate).

GOOD BUYS

There is a multiplicity of Vitamin E products, all of a very standard quality, and it is impossible to suggest the best buys other than by applying the general principles outlined in the Introduction.

Healthilife and Healthcrafts Ranges
Complete ranges of Vitamin E products from low- to high-strength formulae to meet all requirements.

Ephynal Range (10 – 200mg) (ROCHE)
This is also comprehensive.

Blackmore's Range
A range of Vitamin E supplements using natural-source Vitamin E in a variety of strengths. The range comes in both capsules and tablets, the tablets being chewable and suitable for vegetarians, but not for Vegans. They also produce a Vitamin E cream made from natural sources. There is little to suggest that this is therapeutic.

See also: **Glossary; Selenium; Vitamins A and C; Acne; Artery Problems; Cancer; Cataract; Diabetes; Dysmenorrhoea; Fibrocystic Breast Disease; Gall Bladder Problems; Immunodepression; Menopausal Problems; Menorrhagia; PMS.**

ZINC

ZINC, an essential micronutrient or trace element, is involved in more than 80 enzyme systems in the body, and is part of the structure of cell walls. About 60 per cent of the body's zinc is in our muscles and 30 per cent is lodged in our bones. The total amount of zinc in our bodies is about 2g.

Doctors were experimenting with zinc salts as medicines in the 19th century. In the days before phenobarbitone and other anticonvulsant drugs were developed to control epilepsy, mega doses of zinc were found most effective in releasing patients from their recurrent fits. Zinc was also 'promoted' at this time for the treatment of a disease that is still very much with us, anorexia nervosa.

One of the curious things about the history of nutrition is that the veterinary profession so often seems to point the therapeutic finger first in the direction in which the doctors should be looking. A nasty disease of pigs known as porcine psoriasis used to cost pig raisers a lot of money, but in 1955 vets discovered that it could be prevented by adding zinc to pig food. A few years later veterinary surgeons linked a disease of the thymus gland in Friesian cattle with zinc deficiency. This problem, too, was readily cured by zinc supplementation, and because the thymus gland in all animals is closely connected with immunity, a link between zinc and the vital forces of the immune system was forged.

Strangely, the first time that zinc was closely linked to a human disease in recent medical history was when it was discovered that a rare but serious skin disease in young babies, called acrodermatitis enteropathica could be completely cured by zinc supplementation. Previously such babies had frequently to be hospitalised and often died. This new knowledge led to a general awakening of medical interest in zinc and well over 2,500 scientific papers have been published on zinc in medicine over the last few years. Professor Bryce-Smith, probably the foremost expert on zinc metabolism, now lists a formidable array of symptoms in which zinc deficiency may be involved.

The list below is adapted from his book *The Zinc Solution*, co-written with Liz Hodgkinson (Century Arrow, 1986).

Signs and Symptoms of Zinc Deficiency

- Impaired taste and smell
- Pica (craving for peculiar foods, common in pregnancy)
- Growth retardation
- Hypogonadism (immature sexual organs) in males
- Impotence (particularly in kidney dialysis patients)
- Depression, mood changes, impaired concentration
- Intention tremor (a tremor of the hands occurring only during active movements)
- Nystagmus (flickering eyes)
- Speech impairment
- Jitteriness
- Photophobia, night blindness, blepharitis (inflammation of the eyelids)
- Several skin diseases
- Whitlows
- Poor nail growth
- Poor hair growth or alopecia
- Delayed wound healing
- Diarrhoea
- Anorexia and bulimia nervosa
- Subfertility (oligospermia) in males
- Subnormal birth weight and subnormal head circumference in new-born babies

- Spina bifida (in some animals)
- Hepatic encephalopathy (mental disorders caused by the effect of alcoholism on the liver)
- Increased susceptibility to infection
- Acrodermatitis enteropathica
- Acne (some types)
- Stretch marks on skin

Of course, many of these conditions can have other causes as well, but the list of zinc-deficiency possibilities as far as ill-health is concerned have encouraged even very conservative doctors to consider zinc deficiency when faced with an unusual symptom complex.

Do You Need Supplementation?

Most of us probably do not ingest enough zinc in our diets. The average daily intake in the West is less than 10mg, whereas the amount recommended for adults by the US National Academy of Science is 15mg per day.

Those undergoing variable types of stress, trauma or hormonal upheaval can quickly become zinc-deficient and need supplementation. Athletes can become depleted of zinc through sweating.

However, you can easily test for yourself whether or not you are deficient in zinc. This test also comes from Professor Bryce-Smith's book, *The Zinc Solution*.

THE ZINC DEFICIENCY TEST

Get your local pharmacist to make a test solution by dissolving 1 gram of zinc sulphate heptahydrate ($ZnSO_4.7H_2O$) in 1 litre (1¾ pints) of distilled water. Tap water is not recommended as the solution tends to give a slight precipitate on standing. Responses to tasting 5 – 10 millilitres – that is, 1 – 2 teaspoons – of this solution normally place the tasters into one of the following four categories:

1. No specific taste or other sensation is noticed, even after the solution has been kept in the mouth for about 10 seconds. (Some people even find a solution of twice the above strength to be tasteless.)

2. No immediate taste noted, but after a few seconds a slight taste variously described as 'dry', 'mineral', 'furry' or (more rarely) 'sweet' develops.

3. A definite though not unpleasant taste is noted almost immediately, and tends to intensify with time.

4. A strong and unpleasant taste is noted immediately. The subject normally grimaces.

If the response is in either of the first two categories – and especially the first – there is likely to be a favourable response to zinc supplements. These may be discontinued or reduced when responses move up to categories 3 or 4.

— FOOD SOURCES —

Red meat (especially beef); fish (especially oysters, shellfish); wholegrain cereals; legumes. The availability from cereals may be reduced because their phytic acid content binds calcium, iron and zinc, so that the body cannot absorb them. If a bread is yeast-leavened, however, this lessens the binding effect of the phytic acid.

Vegetables contain moderate amounts of zinc provided they are grown on soil with a reasonable zinc content.

One of the worrying things about zinc as a nutrient is that it is relatively poorly absorbed from food. Alcohol, smoking and high-fibre diets inhibit absorption, as do soya proteins, coffee, cows' milk, cheese and celery. Zinc 'promoters' include Vitamins A and D and citrus fruits.

Committed vegetarians and those on relatively meat-free diets are at potential risk because it is comparatively easy to 'boil out' zinc from vegetables. A diet composed largely of processed foods will also be low in zinc.

ACNE AND ZINC

The first possible connection between acne and zinc was made by a Swedish dermatologist in 1973. His subject was a male teenager who had suffered from the skin disorder acrodermatitis enteropathica as a child, and was now suffering from severe acne. After zinc supplementation, the boy showed rapid improvement. Further zinc trials showed a marked decrease in control groups of severe pustular and papular acne.

However, although further studies have not proved the relationship between zinc and acne so decisively as that between zinc and acrodermatitis enteropathica, it is worthwhile trying zinc as an aid in acne management. Puberty, when acne more usually strikes, is a time of much stress, of hormonal upheaval and rapid growth. Zinc is needed for growth, and it can also help restore hormone balances, but it can be leached from the body through stress.

ANOREXIA AND BULIMIA NERVOSA AND ZINC

It was Professor Derek Bryce-Smith who first recognised the re-lationship between anorexia, bulimia and zinc. In these 'dieting' diseases, many of the physical and mental symptoms appeared to him to be exactly what one might expect of a zinc deficiency – primarily poor appetite and loss of senses of taste and smell.

Knowing that the British diet was already seriously deficient in zinc, and that some people are poor absorbers, he found that many anorexia and bulimia sufferers did indeed appear to have a subnormal ability to absorb dietary zinc from the gut. Most of the patients were teenage girls as well, already undergoing the stresses of adolescence, exams, the desire to be slim and to be liked, and these would in themselves further deplete the body of zinc.

The results of supplementation, as reported in his book, appear little short of miraculous. Within weeks in some cases, severe sufferers had regained some weight and, more important, had lost their phobias about food, and had become more mentally and socially balanced. Within a month or so many anorexics and bulimics taking the zinc deficiency test (see page 150–1) had progressed from category 1 to category 4.

BALDING, SCALP AND HAIR PROBLEMS AND ZINC

Low levels of zinc in the body have been associated with conditions that lead to hair loss. Zinc has been used with some success to treat alopecia areata, a disease of sudden baldness, as well as hair loss associated with excessive scalp dryness.

BED SORES AND ZINC

Zinc supplementation has been shown to speed up the healing of wounds. The stress of the wound, whether surgical, accidental or the skin damage of bed sores, can cause zinc to be lost from the body. Zinc ointments are good, but an oral dosage has been particularly effective, sometimes halving the time of wound healing after surgical operations. Some researchers believe that supplementation *in advance of* surgery can also help.

COLDS AND ZINC

Zinc would appear to have antiviral and antibacterial properties, because of its association with the thymus gland and the lymphatic system. These are responsible for effective mobilisation of the body's defensive white blood cells.

Once again, Professor Derek Bryce-Smith is the zinc proponent. He refers us to a US study group of the elderly, between the ages of 60 and 97, who were given supplements of 35mg of extra zinc daily for four weeks, and who subsequently showed increased resistance to all kinds of infection, including colds. He also refers to a study by a team working from the University of Texas that looked into the effect of lozenges containing 23mg of zinc gluconate that, if sucked by common cold sufferers, reduced the duration of cold symptoms by about a week.

As might be expected, neither of these reports was substantial enough to impress the scientific community, and they are mainly looked upon as interesting examples of folk medicine in action. Nevertheless, in the face of virtually nothing specific in the way of medicines being available to 'cure a cold', something as simple and safe as zinc would seem to earn a place in a good health food-guide.

HERPES AND ZINC

Zinc has been shown to inhibit the replication of the virus which causes herpes.

An Australian dermatologist gave his patients with recurrent herpes Vitamin C 200mg and zinc sulphate 100mg twice daily for six weeks. He found that this therapy either prevented the herpes completely, reduced its severity or, curiously, produced a violent herpes eruption that was followed by subsequent immunity to recurrent herpes, provided therapy was continued. Surprisingly perhaps, this simple therapy has not been subsequently explored.

The likelihood that zinc is in some way helpful in the management of recurrent herpes is underlined in an impressive double blind trial report in which the zinc was applied as a simple ointment (Ung Zinc Sulph 0.05%) or mixed with lithium succinate and Vitamin E. In this trial, which involved 200 patients (a mixture of Type I and II herpes infection victims), there was a quick relief of symptoms and rapid healing. The active preparation significantly reduced the duration of pain symptoms from seven to four days.

VARICOSE ULCERS AND ZINC

As with bed sores, zinc has proved itself invaluable in speeding up varicose ulcer healing.

Professor Derek Bryce-Smith quotes a pioneer study carried out in Australia in which ten varicose ulcer patients were given zinc sulphate tablets three times a day or a placebo tablet in a single blind trial. Patients taking the zinc had an ulcer healing rate that was three times faster than that observed in the placebo trials. Subsequently another single blinded trial of 27 patients, which also looked at serum zinc levels, showed that zinc-treated patients healed faster as their blood zinc levels became normal.

Dosage, Side Effects and Contraindications

For all but the most serious cases, a supplement providing 8 – 15mg of zinc per day should be sufficient.

Zinc can cause gastrointestinal upset. If too much zinc is taken, chronic indigestion can result. Doses of over 50mg per day may predispose towards the development of anaemia; long-term doses of the same size can interfere with copper metabolism. Very large doses of zinc – in the region of 2g per day – are acutely toxic and produce nausea, vomiting and fever.

Zinc supplements should not be combined with tetracycline antibiotics or be prescribed to patients suffering from kidney failure.

The values and recommended dosages I have given for zinc refer to elemental zinc. However, many supplements contain zinc in the form of amino acid chelate or zinc gluconate, because it is thought by some that absorption is greater when zinc is taken in these forms. Remember that 15mg of zinc gluconate or amino acid chelated zinc do not actually supply 15g of elemental zinc: with amino acid-chelated zinc, for example, the 25mg is made up of the zinc *plus* its accompanying chelate.

Dietary Reference Values for Zinc, mg per day

Age	LRNI		EAR		RNI	
11–14 yr	5.3		7.0		9.0	
	Males	Females	Males	Females	Males	Females
15 + yr	5.5	4.0	7.3	5.5	9.5	7.0

Additional amounts to be added to pre-pregnancy DRVs		
Lactating women:	0–4 months	+ 6.0
	4 + months	+ 2.5

GOOD BUYS

Bio Zinc (BLACKMORE'S)
Contains 40mg of zinc amino acid chelate, (which provides

4mg elemental zinc. This product is sugar-free, and contains no wheat, yeast, cornstarch, milk derivatives, gluten, preservatives, artificial colours or flavours, or animal substances, and is therefore suitable for vegetarians and Vegans.

Synergistic Zinc (QUEST)

This particular brand is called 'synergistic' because it also contains copper and Vitamin A, both of which help in the absorption of the zinc. It contains 133mg of zinc amino acid chelate, which provides 20mg of elemental zinc. This product is also useful for people who suffer from allergies to wheat and to milk products. It is free from artificial preservatives, colours and flavours, added starch, sucrose, lactose or salt, yeast, wheat or gluten. It is suitable for vegetarians.

Food Supplement Company Range

Zinc contains 30mg of zinc gluconate which provides 4mg of elemental zinc.

Zinc Picolinate is a zinc supplement of 30mg of elemental zinc.

Zinc Lozenges and Vitamin C and peppermint contain 25mg of zinc gluconate which provides 3.5mg of elemental zinc per lozenge. This form of zinc is used at the onset of a cold or sore throat.

Healthilife Range

Zinc contains 40mg of amino acid-chelated zinc, which provides 4mg of elemental zinc in an amino acid-chelated capsule.

Mega Zinc Lozenges each contain 80mg of zinc gluconate, which provides 11.2mg of elemental zinc and 50mg of Vitamin C. These are an excellent source of zinc for those who have trouble swallowing tablets.

Cantassium

Cantassium have a zinc product in their range which contains 10mg of zinc.

See also: **Acne; Anorexia Nervosa; Balding, Scalp and Hair Problems; Bed Sores; Colds; Herpes; Varicose Veins, Ulcers and Haemorrhoids.**

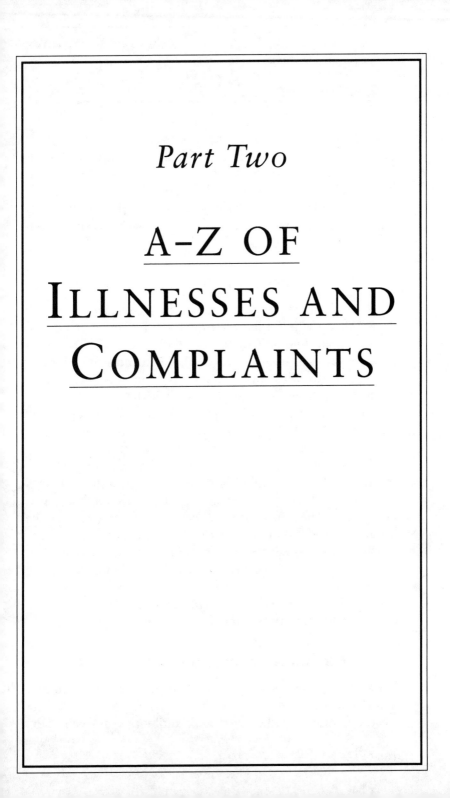

Part Two

A–Z OF
ILLNESSES AND
COMPLAINTS

ACNE

ACNE is the commonest disease of the skin, and if you are a teenager, you will probably experience some degree of it. Girls are affected at an earlier age than boys, but it is the latter that the disease tends to affect more severely. The chances are that you will be clear of acne by your early twenties, but in 6 per cent of sufferers the disease can persist up to between the ages of 25 and 40.

Signs and Symptoms

Fundamentally, the disease is caused by a blockage of the tiny duct (called the pilo-sebaceous duct) of the grease gland that lubricates the fine hair of the face and back. This blockage causes a blackhead to develop, the 'blackness' of which is nothing to do with dirt but with pigment (melanin) being leached out from the hair. These blackheads can become infected, and can spread and develop into spots, cysts and boils. The skin is tender and inflamed and, in severe cases of acne, can be permanently damaged and scarred.

Why this blockage of the duct happens remains rather a medical mystery. Probably hormone changes around puberty make natural hair grease just that much more solid than it was before. For acne is primarily a disease which is triggered by the hormones, and it is at puberty that these are most active. Acne can flare up at other times of hormonal change; women can have increased trouble pre-menstrually and, rarely, at the menopause.

Excessive intake of iodine can produce or aggravate acne. In such cases the culprit is often an iodine-rich cough mixture.

Orthodox Medical Management

Doctors and skin specialists first of all advise careful skin care and cleanliness, and mild skin-peeling agents. Severe cases are treated with skin abrasives and antibiotics as well. Sex-hormone manipulation using similar drugs to those present in the Pill helps in some severe and persistent acne cases in females. Ultraviolet light and/or sunshine help many victims of both sexes at the (later) expense of premature skin ageing and an increased risk of skin cancer. (But sometimes acne is *aggravated* by sunshine.)

Although acne sufferers have been denied chocolate as part of acne management, modern clinical trials have indicated that chocolate eating has no effect on the course of acne. It is wisest, however, particularly during puberty, to avoid over-processed foods, fatty foods, and those containing a lot of sugar.

Good Health-Food Management

ZINC AND ACNE

There are several zinc preparations available in tablet form that have won a firm reputation in the treatment of acne. However, quite rarely zinc causes dyspepsia. It should only be taken under medical supervision in patients suffering from kidney disease. It should not be taken if tetracyclines are also being taken. Otherwise it is a safe and useful dietary supplement in acne cases. The possibility that zinc might be helpful in acne was suggested when it was discovered that acne sufferers had considerably less zinc in their blood, hair and nails than acne-free patients.

Trial evidence supports the use of zinc supplementation in acne management. The best results occur when a relatively substantial (but quite safe) dose of zinc is taken over a period of 6 to 12 weeks (50mg of elemental zinc thrice daily or 135mg of zinc sulphate daily). It is sensible to consult your pharmacist as to the most appropriate preparation available, and to purchase only a small quantity to start with, in case you are one of those who develop a 'zinc dyspepsia'.

SELENIUM, VITAMIN E AND ACNE

Selenium is a micronutrient that is, for several reasons, usually taken combined with Vitamin E. Taken in DRV (dietary reference value) doses, selenium preparations are completely safe. An observational and an experimental study are the basis of the use of selenium and Vitamin E in Acne. (Toxic levels of selenium are reached only at approximately 100 times the usual recommended dose.) There seem to be no adverse reactions to DRVs of selenium/Vitamin E preparations, and no problems relative to other medication.

VITAMIN B₆ (PYRIDOXINE) AND ACNE

There is some evidence that Vitamin B_6 can help alleviate the type of acne that appears at period times.

GOOD BUYS

★*Gold Standard*
Zinc products, e.g. Zinc One-A-Day (HEALTHCRAFTS) and Zinc Gluconate (HEALTHRITE).

Useful
● Selenium and Vitamin E products, e.g. Selenium-ACE (WASSEN) ● When associated with PMS, any Vitamin B_6 product.

See also: **Selenium; Vitamin E; Vitamin B₆; Zinc; Menopause; PMS.**

AGEING

RANDOM ageing is what happens to all of us, you might say. But this is to some extent under our control. The easiest example of random ageing in action is seen in what happens if we expose our skin to high doses of sunshine for longer than is good for us. You can see this sort of ageing if you look at the faces of middle-aged people who live in Australia or California, where there once was a cult of sun worship without sunscreens. Constant over-exposure to ultraviolet light destroys the skin's subcutaneous elastic tissue, and the skin looks old much too soon for its chronological biological status. (X-rays do the same sort of thing to skin, as do certain chemicals and pharmaceuticals, notably some hydrocortisone ointments.)

But perhaps the most prevalent ageing reaction is one that occurs as a result of the reaction on our bodies of atomic and molecular agents known as *oxidants* or *free radicals* (see Glossary). These can be beneficial but, when they become unstable, can cause considerable damage to tissue and general body health. To hold the degenerative diseases of ageing at bay, the ravages of the free radicals must be checked, and this is where the *anti*oxidants (Vitamins A, beta-carotene, C and E and the micronutrient selenium) come in. If the body has a good bank of antioxidants at its disposal, the destructive action of the free radicals is inhibited.

Closely associated with the action of free radicals in ageing is the phenomenon of *cross linking*. What is it that old leather, stale bread, superannuated windscreen wipers, 'elderly' plastic-covered garden furniture, the skin on the back of your hand or your forehead, and perhaps even the internal tissues of your blood vessels, have in common? The answer is the same ageing process, brought about by that same cross linking.

Basically, all these phenomena are evidence of a biochemical process in which body proteins lose their flexibility. Subsequently the biological blueprints that are characterised in DNA and RNA then become 'blurred' too, giving what would seem to be faulty instructions to cells, particularly to cell proteins.

It is thought that cross linking damage to DNA is one of the principal factors in ageing. As we grow older the whole body becomes stiffer, less 'elastic', less resilient and less agile. In the same way as your old windscreen wiper rubber no longer conforms to the curve of your car windscreen and starts to screech as it smudges rather than wipes, our tissues at a molecular level fall foul of cross linking, too.

One way to get a rough and ready guide as to where you are at the present moment relative to cross linking in your body is to place your hand palm down on a table and lift a 'pinch' of the skin on the back of your hand on hold it there for 5 seconds on

In a young person, the pinch obliterates itself in seconds on release. In older people the ridge of skin distortion takes much longer, and just how much longer demonstrates just how far cross linking has aged your body.

This little experiment would be a depressing reminder of our ultimate morbidity and mortality if it were not just for one thing. We do have at our disposal today the antioxidants that delay the process of cross linking.

Ageing really describes Nature's seemingly unkind obsolescence system in action. (A quick and ready example of biological ageing in action is the menopause, the cessation of fertility, which occurs right on time, in the majority of women, around the age of 50.)

Signs and Symptoms

It can seem as if everything in the body is gradually packing up: bones and joints become less mobile; memory, sight and hearing are diminished. Some of the changes are not directly related to physical health, such as the colour changes of hair and the wrinkling of the skin.

It is important to remember that very few people die of old age itself, but of a disease process. If disease processes can be prevented, checked or ameliorated in any way, then ageing can be much less traumatic.

Orthodox Medical Management

This consists largely of common-sense exhortations to eat well, to take exercise, and generally to look after oneself as well as one can. Illnesses are treated promptly, and it is interesting that most of these are illnesses to which everyone, even people much younger, is prone. One problem doctors find is that old people tend to feel that their complaint or pain is all to do with their age and do not seek medical advice *soon* enough, and also do not bother about *taking* that advice, feeling there's no point in doing so.

Good Health-Food Management

Because of the newly discovered and appreciated properties of the antioxidants, the ageing process can be controlled to some extent, if not reversed.

SELENIUM AND AGEING

Alan Lewis, the editor of *Here's Health*, made a small beginning as a medical geographer when he started a study of selenium and the elderly. In East Anglia, and particularly around Upper Sheringham, he found there were two to three times as many people over the age of 75 than in the country as a whole. Living in an agricultural area, most of these people grew a lot of their own food; the soil was also rich in selenium.

He then undertook a world trip to meet as many very senior citizens as possible and to assess their selenium intakes. His multinational team of Russian, French and US scientists found in one Russian village of 1,200 inhabitants, there were 71 men and 110 women between the ages of 81 and 90. Nineteen were over 90, and there were several centenarians. Racially these folk were Abkazian nomads, who lived mostly on fruit, beans and root vegetables well-flavoured with garlic, which is a selenium-rich diet. Sugar was never eaten, and meat-eating was rare. This added up to a low-fat, high-fibre diet and, again, one rich in natural mineral sources, especially selenium.

The Hunzas of Pakistan are another group who has more than a fair share of aged, yet very active, citizens. They also eat a vegetable diet, rich in pulses and low in meat.

Comparing the Norfolk 'golden oldies' with those in Russia and Pakistan, there are several similarities, the most striking of which is lack of industrialisation and a habit of eating a lot of home-grown vegetable produce. But the main dramatic similarity is that by some sort of geographical accident they all also enjoy living in a selenium-rich soil area, and so get a good intake of selenium from their locally-grown food.

This connection is interesting enough in itself, but when you consider the degenerative diseases which selenium and the other antioxidants are said to help – among them artery and cardiac problems, arthritis, rheumatism and cancer – it can be seen that selenium supplementation can have a very positive part to play. As well as potentially preventing many of the diseases our flesh is heir to, it can contribute to each of us looking, feeling and staying 'younger'.

GINSENG AND AGEING

It is primarily in China – where ginseng has long been valued – that the plant is associated with benefits for the ageing. However, it is probably its 'adaptogen' properties (see page 50) – which selenium shares – which are the practical explanation of how ginseng helps the body and mind to cope with stress or medical problems, whatever it might be. Ageing can be full of unacknowledged terrors, both physical and emotional, and anything which could help alleviate these is worth trying.

POLLEN AND AGEING

If the curative powers of royal jelly seem, despite their famous and passionate proponents, to be less than scientifically possible, this is not so clear so far as pollen supplementation is concerned. In tests on elderly people (see page 90), pollen was shown to be of considerable benefit.

COENZYME Q10 AND ALZHEIMER'S DISEASE

There have been many studies which favourably link CoQ10 and Alzheimer's Disease, the progressive failure of cerebral function which can occur after the age of 50.

GOOD BUYS
- Selenium products, e.g. Selenium-ACE (WASSEN)
- Coenzyme Q10 (HEALTHILIFE, WASSEN).

Worth Trying
- Gingseng • Pollen.

See also: **Alzheimer's Disease; Ginseng; Glossary; Pollen, Propolis and Royal Jelly; Selenium; Vitamins A and C.**

ALCOHOLISM

ALCOHOLISM is a condition of dependence brought about by the consumption of alcohol. Because of geographical differences about the amounts of alcohol that are socially acceptable, whether or not someone is an alcoholic is not easy to define. However, the condition becomes a disease if the need to drink is so urgent that it adversely affects the lifestyle of the drinker, his or her sleep patterns, and leads to stresses and difficulties both at home and work.

In a nutritional sense, heavy alcohol use displaces other, more nutritious foods in the diet, and impairs the absorption and metabolism of nutrients. It also fosters obesity.

Orthodox and Good Health-Food Management

Stopping drinking, and following a good diet, plus psychological guidance in the form of counselling, are the primary ways in which to manage alcoholism. There are a few relevant health foods, a supplement of which may help alleviate some of the physical symptoms resulting from heavy drinking.

MAGNESIUM AND ALCOHOLISM

Alcohol, even a moderate social amount, is magnesuretic – it allows some of the body's meagre stores of magnesium to be pumped out of the body tissues through the kidneys in urine. (Zinc can disappear in much the same way.) This encourages a lack of magnesium balance which can result in palpitations of the heart (which in itself is reliant on good stores of magnesium).

However, that is not the end of the story. There is a wealth of undisputed medical evidence that chronic alcoholics develop severe symptoms of tachycardia (palpitations) when they are being 'dried out'. These alcohol tachycardias are sometimes found to be associated with low blood magnesium.

167

EVENING PRIMROSE OIL AND ALCOHOLISM

Alcohol inteferes with linolenic acid metabolism. Some alcohol detoxification centres advise evening primrose oil supplements for alcoholics.

THE B VITAMINS AND ALCOHOLISM

Many of the clinical conditions associated with alcoholism are related to a Vitamin B deficiency, especially B_1 (thiamin). (Beri-beri is the most noted thiamin deficiency disease, and although rare now in the countries in which it was endemic – caused by diets consisting mostly of polished rice – it is occasionally seen in heavy drinkers.) Wernicke-Korsakoff syndrome is a serious disorder of the central nervous system occurring in alcoholism. In orthodox medicine, there is often a good response to B_1 supplementation.

Heavy drinking can also bring about a folate deficiency, and folate deficiency at the time of a baby's conception is linked with neural-tube defect disease, especially spina bifida. This is why pregnant women are advised to avoid alcoholic drinks.

GOOD BUYS

● Magnesium OK (WASSEN) ● Any multivitamin B preparation.

See also: **Birth defects; B Vitamins; Evening Primrose Oil; Magnesium.**

ALLERGY

AN allergy is a hypersensitive reaction to substances called antigens, which are foreign to the body and to which the body is exposed in everyday life. When antigens cause the exaggerated reactions of allergy, they are known as allergens, and they include pollen, animal hair, house dust mites, adhesives, cement, nickel, foods such as shellfish and eggs, and food additives such as MSG (monosodium glutamate). Basically you can be allergic to almost anything!

An allergic reaction can be an instant thing – to a sting, say – or it can take years to develop: for instance to the nickel in your wristwatch or earring, or to the chromium in cement (this can take some 20 years plus). It is the battle between allergen and antibodies (the body's defence system) which causes the sufferer's allergic ailments.

Perhaps the most extraordinary feature as far as allergy is concerned is that infection and the activities of our central nervous system can be involved in an allergic reaction too. Psychological upsets can trigger off an allergic response, but only if other allergens, or allergy triggers, are around.

This whole complex process can be simplified by looking at allergy as being triggered in three possible ways – sometimes represented as a circle or 'cake'.

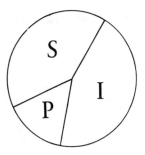

Sensitivity substance

Infection

Psychological

} relative sizes of slices are very variable

The 'slices' of this allergy cake can vary enormously in the contribution they make to an allergic reaction. For instance, sensitising substances, and especially pollens, make up most of the 'cake' in hayfever, in which infection and psychological factors are involved minimally. Looking at your allergy as a 'multifactorial' condition can make it easier to cope with. (But psychological effects *can* trigger off hayfever: some people develop it while reading the pollen count in newspapers when they are half a mile away from pollen in a city underground!)

Signs and Symptoms

The nature of the allergic reaction varies considerably, according to the individual, the allergen itself, and where and how the allergen enters the body. The skin can redden, become irritated and itchy, and develop a rash or weals. If the nose is affected, the sufferer will sneeze and produce mucus. The eyes can weep and swell. (A combination of nose and eye allergic reaction is hayfever, caused by grass or tree pollen in the air.) Reaction in the lungs can cause asthmatic attacks. If a food is ingested to which a sufferer is allergic, stomach pain and diarrhoea can be accompanied by a skin reaction.

Orthodox Medical Management

This is generally brought about by antihistamine tablets, steroid ointments, tablets or injections. Sometimes specific anti-allergy agents containing sodium cromoglycate are prescribed. De-sensitisation injections are less used these days.

Good Health Food Management

The common allergy diseases that health foods can help with are hayfever, allergic rhinitis, eczema and allergic dermatitis, and food allergies, particularly to monosodium glutamate (MSG). This substance is widely used as a flavour improver, and is the prime cause of the 'Chinese restaurant syndrome'.

The relatively high incidence of side effects in conventional therapy for allergy, and the tendency that exists for overdosage (following the seductively spectacular effects of initial therapy), has led to an interest in the introduction of health-food-type management. If you suffer from food allergy, particularly to MSG, it is worthwhile trying the effect of pyridoxine (Vitamin B_6) in a dosage of 50mg per day for 12 weeks. This often cures the sensitivity but the side effects of B_6 dosage should be borne in mind (see page 126).

If you suffer from an eczema-type reaction on your skin to various or individual substances, evening primrose oil can often help. It can also help infantile eczema, which is often an allergic reaction to cows' milk.

GOOD BUYS

● For food allergy, pyridoxine (B_6) 50mg products ● For skin problems, evening primrose oil products.

See also: **Vitamin B_6; Evening Primrose Oil; Eczema and Allergic Dermatitis; Hayfever and Allergic Rhinitis; Irritable Bowel Syndrome.**

ALOPECIA

See Balding and Scalp and Hair Problems.

ALZHEIMER'S DISEASE

ALZHEIMER'S Disease, or AD, is the term now used for both senile and pre-senile dementia. It is diagnosed by its history (progressive failure of cerebral function) and characteristic CT (computerised tomography) scan. It has to be differentiated from 20 or so dementing diseases, because many of these respond to medical treatement (e.g. hypothyroidism [a disease in which the thyroid is defective in some degree], pellagra [caused by a Vitamin B_2 deficiency], and various poisonings), whereas AD does not. Cynical doctors like the term AD, and say that if you can remember how to spell Alzheimer's, you have not got it!

The basic cause of AD is unknown.

Signs and Symptoms

The condition is seldom seen below the age of 50, and a familial tendency is unusual. Memory failure, progressive intellectural decline and apathy characterise the AD victim. Sometimes symptoms suggest the part of the brain most profoundly affected, for example speech problems and defects. Sometimes AD is heralded by a profound depression. The disease progresses at a variable rate. Some victims develop a stoop and an expressionless face. Epileptic fits can complicate AD.

Orthodox Medical Management

None, other than domestic or residential care (after the exclusion of other treatable neurological conditions).

The fact that excessive aluminium exposure in animals and memory loss in adults is sometimes associated with small increases in serum aluminium has led to contemporary interest in an anti-aluminium therapy and the avoidance of aluminium kitchenware in food preparation, but no convincing experimental evidence exists that such manoeuvres have any effect on progression in AD, and several medical conditions increase brain aluminium without producing AD. Research involving fluoride could be interesting (see page 44).

Nevertheless, a geographical association does exist between Alzheimer's Disease and levels of aluminium in water supplies, and there is a hypothesis that silicon in the diet may reduce the bio-availability (see Glossary) of aluminium. Dietary supplements of silicon do not seem to be prevalent at the moment. Food sources rich in silicon include alfalfa, cabbage, lettuce, onions, dark greens, kelp and milk. Food processing relentlessly removes silicon from food. (Milled flour contains only 2 per cent of its original silicon.)

Exactly how such a seemingly inert substance as silicon could effect a complex neurological disease such as AD would seem to be puzzling, but work carried out by Klaus Schwarz and Edith Carlisle in the 1970s linked an atherogenic diet (i.e. one that is liable to predispose the development of atheroma or the hardening of the arteries) with low arterial tissue levels of silicon, and showed that low silicon in animal skin was associated with premature skin ageing.

When one considers that the central nervous system and the skin develop embryologically from the same cells, and that many of the symptoms of Alzheimer's Disease are similar to those exhibited in senile athero-sclerotic dementia, silicon and mental health may well be quite closely linked.

Good Health-Food Management

Due to the paucity of effective measurement, attention is paid to methods of treatment that 'could be helpful'.

COENZYME Q10 AND ALZHEIMER'S DISEASE

The most recent of these helpful possibilities is Coenzyme Q10 or CoQ10, which has the capacity to restore and improve many functions which are lessened in the AD victim.

VITAMINS AND ALZHEIMER'S DISEASE

Perhaps more significant at the present state of the therapeutic game, is the long-overdue realisation that demented people are more likely than others to be nutritionally deficient. This has led to observational studies that have demonstrated improvement occurring in AD victims being treated with Vitamins B_{12}, C, D, E, beta-carotene and folate, or folic acid.

GOOD BUYS

• Vitamin supplements with Vitamins B_{12}, C, D, E, beta-carotene and folate, especially if demonstrably deficient • Coenzyme Q_{10} and Vitamin E (WASSEN) • Alfalfa and kelp products may have a useful prophylactic function, for example Kelp (HEALTHCRAFTS) and Wild Ocean Kelp (LANES) • A silicon product is marketed by Health Innovations Ltd as Kervran's Silica (extracted from natural horsetail); although promoted as a nail and hair improver, it could well be helpful in countering the symptoms of Alzheimer's Disease.

See also: **Ageing; Coenzyme Q10; Vitamins A, B, C, D and E.**

ANAEMIA

A DISEASE in which haemoglobin (the oxygen carrier in the blood) is reduced. In practice, the diagnosis of anaemia groups together a large number of diseases. By far the commonest type of anaemia is a nutritional deficiency disease brought about by the body's constant need for iron, a mineral normally provided from everyday diet, not being fully met.

Major sources of iron in food come from meat, eggs, milk, flour and green vegetables. The body is very clever as far as storing iron is concerned, and iron absorption becomes much more efficient when iron stores in the body are low, so why do we get anaemic?

Look at iron-deficiency anaemia as if it were a bath full of water. A bath of water will tend to empty gradually by evaporation unless it is periodically topped up by, say, a dripping tap. We all lose iron from our bodies all of the time

(0.5 – 1mg per day) in our faeces, skin, urine and sweat. Women also lose an extra 0.7mg of iron each day that they menstruate; women with very heavy periods become anaemic because they just cannot absorb enough iron from their food to compensate for this blood loss. Both sexes quite rarely get anaemia through various blood-loss diseases – piles or bleeding peptic ulcers, for instance – or because the blood-forming organ in the body becomes diseased. There is also evidence that many people are 'poor absorbers' of iron. Small children and the elderly, for instance, have special difficulty in absorbing iron from the diet.

The causes of iron-deficiency anaemia are therefore due to 1) not eating enough iron-rich food; 2) poor absorption; or 3) increased demands for iron, due to blood loss.

Signs and Symptoms

The symptoms that suggest you might be anaemic are fatigue, feeling easily tired, headaches, or faintness. Breathlessness, chest or leg pain on exertion and palpitations may occur, too. Because these symptoms are common to many medical problems and, indeed, may be present in normal people, it is important always for an accurate diagnosis of anaemia to be made by means of a blood test. This will not only diagnose the exact cause of the anaemia but will also indicate its severity and dictate treatment. In persistent anaemia, victims notice that their nails and hair are brittle and often their tongue or mouth gets sore and they have problems with swallowing.

The signs and symptoms of anaemia often indicate its severity. A doctor can diagnose a severe case from the other side of the street. Minor degrees need careful blood testing.

Orthodox Medical and Good Health-Food Management

If anaemia is shown to be simply nutritional, it can be cured by 1) stopping the blood loss (for example, excessive menstruation); and 2) increasing the iron intake in food. This

175

is unlikely to restore the balance, and the taking of iron supplements is usually necessary. Enough iron has to be taken not only to replace iron in the blood but also replenish the body's diminished iron stores. The most economical and efficient way to do this is by taking simple iron preparations such as ferrous sulphate or ferrous gluconate in a dose of 300mg per day. (However, iron therapy is associated with side effects in many people, see page 72.)

Once a nutritional anaemia has been corrected, either by medical treatment or by supplementation with iron-rich health foods, it would seem to be sensible to supplement the daily diet permanently by means of a health food containing meaningful amounts of iron. It is easier to maintain 'iron positive health' once it has been obtained than to remedy an anaemia.

GOOD BUYS

Generally speaking the cheapest iron preparation available is as efficient as the dearest in treating anaemia, although some experts believe that iron plus Vitamin C preparations are better than iron on its own (C aids absorption of the iron). If any iron preparation causes nausea, indigestion or constipation, try halving the dose. If this does not help, consult a doctor.

If you opt for an 'iron plus' health food, check the packet to see that its daily dosage contains 100 per cent of your daily iron requirement. Good health foods give you this information.

★ *Gold Standard*
● Ferrous iron products available from chemist shops (see page 73).

Useful
● Synergistic Iron (QUEST) ● Blackstrap Molasses Iron (FSC)
● Genesis (WASSEN) ● Aminochel Iron (HEALTHCRAFTS)
● Minadex (SEVEN SEAS).

Probably ineffective
● Iron-fortified cereals.

See also: **Menorrhagia; Tiredness and Fatigue; Iron; Vitamin C.**

ANOREXIA AND BULIMIA NERVOSA

VARIOUS surveys suggest that between one and ten females for each 100,000 young women in the population between the ages of 15 and 34 are victims of these eating disorders. The most common age group to suffer is the 16- to 17-year-old. It seldom appears after the age of 55, and is rare in males.

Signs and Symptoms

Symptoms include a weight that is 25 per cent below the standard weight for age and height, an absence of the menstrual cycle, an intense wish to be thin and a morbid fear of fatness. Usually it is a disorder of adolescence in which there has been a previous history of chubbiness or fatness and a relentless pursuit of weight loss. Victims usually have a distorted image of their body size, they eat very little, particularly of carbohydrate. In about 20 per cent of cases, a cessation of the periods precedes the weight loss, and there is usually a lack of any sexual interest. Sometimes there is evidence of an unusual amount of fine body hair (lanugo). Some cases are characterised by periods of binge eating, self-induced vomiting and laxative abuse, in which case the diagnostic term used is *bulimia nervosa*. Sometimes bulimia patients abuse slimming drugs and diuretic drugs to bring about a weight loss.

Bulimia can reach epidemic proportion in closed communities like boarding schools, hostels and university campuses, with rates of 5 – 30 per cent of girls being affected. In addition to the signs and symptoms of anorexia, bulimia sufferers can also suffer from swollen glands in the neck, damaged dental enamel, alcohol dependence, rapid fluctuation in weight, upset rather than absence of menstruation, and personality change. In addition, the self-induced vomiting depletes the body of potassium.

177

Orthodox Medical Management

In many cases this results in hospital admission due to the potential danger associated with these conditions, and concentrates on physical, psychological and family factors. In the case of youngsters many believe that family psychotherapy is essential. In about 30–40 per cent of cases there is a background of childhood sexual abuse. Some psychotherapists believe that the basic cause of this eating disorder is a desire to lose the physical body changes associated with sexual maturity and to return to the less stress-ridden experience of childhood. In bulimia, anti-depressant drugs are often prescribed. Dietary measures to restore electrolyte (potassium and sodium) balance always take pride of place. Many patients need long-term treatment and support (up to three years).

With orthodox treatment 50 per cent of anorexic patients make a complete recovery, 25 per cent have a partial recovery, and the remainder run a chronic course. Mortality may be as high as 10 per cent. In bulimia, prognosis is rather better and about two-thirds of all cases recover and remain well.

Good Health-Food Management

With such a poor showing by orthodox medicine many victims turn to health-food management. This should only be practised against an adequate understanding of the risks of these eating disorders, in which suicide is reported in up to 5 per cent of patients with chronic anorexia nervosa.

POTASSIUM AND BULIMIA NERVOSA

Lowered rates of potassium in the blood can bring about heart-rate disorders, impaired kidney function, and muscular problems. Potassium supplementation should form part of orthodox medical management.

ZINC AND ANOREXIA/BULIMIA NERVOSA

Zinc deficiency is well known to be associated with a lessening of ability to taste and smell: this links these eating disorders with zinc deficiency and the lowered absorption of zinc associated with oral contraceptive usage.

Zinc in any of the proprietary forms should be taken in dosages equivalent to 50mg of zinc sulphate three times a day. Observational and experimental studies using zinc supplementation have provided encouraging results, but no controlled trials are available.

GOOD BUYS

● Zinc Range (HEALTHCRAFTS) ● A good multi-mineral/ multi-vitamin preparation would also seem mandatory, e.g. Genesis (WASSEN).

See also: **Tension and Stress; Potassium; Zinc.**

ARTERY PROBLEMS

THE commonest and most important artery disease is called atherosclerosis (or arteriosclerosis). Commonly this is called hardening of the arteries. Exactly which artery is 'hardened' often gives the name to the actual artery problem, and dictates its signs and symptoms.

Signs and Symptoms

If the coronary arteries are hardened, the chest pain on exertion you can experience is called angina, and perhaps coronary thrombosis may develop. If the leg arteries are hardened, the calf pain on exercise called claudication occurs. Blood vessel disease in the brain can produce stroke illness or dementia. Sometimes the body reacts to artery problems by increasing your blood pressure. This in turn can lead to further problems.

What happens is that the arteries narrow because of the build-up of fatty plaque; if a blood clot forms and blocks the narrowed arteries, blood flow to the heart or brain is interrupted, with serious, occasionally fatal, results.

Orthodox Medical Management

This understandably tends to be tailored to fit the anatomy of the disease if possible, and involves a tremendously wide area of therapy. For example, surgical treatment is often undertaken to replace diseased arteries, and this is becoming commonplace (by-pass surgery). Whether or not the arterial disease is associated with high blood pressure determines whether or not anti-hypertensive drugs are necessary. Many doctors advocate regular small doses of aspirin as a preventative measure. In many cases doctors find themselves involved in trying to cope with advanced arterial disease that might well have been avoidable if preventative measures, such as stopping smoking, taking sensible exercise and not getting obese, had been heeded by the victim.

Dietary Management

All doctors agree that the healthiest diet to prevent atherosclerosis is one in which less than 25 per cent of the calories are derived from fat. But this not the whole story. A concept of 'healthy' and 'unhealthy' fat has evolved. Nutritionally, fats are described in terms of their chemistry as unsaturated or saturated. Saturated fats come from animal sources mostly, and are also present as hydrogenated vegetable fats in certain margarines. These saturated fats are now deemed 'unhealthy'.

When the fat content of any diet is considered, the hidden fats in meat, meat products, pastry, biscuits, etc. must be carefully taken into account. The fact that your body can convert simple sugars and alcohol into unhealthy saturated body fat should always be borne in mind, too. It is pretty crazy to cut all the fat off your chop if you wash it down with a few glasses of wine and ladle sugar on your dessert.

Unfortunately, medical science found itself much more preoccupied with blood cholesterol as an indicator of a liability to develop artery and blood-clotting diseases than in dietary manipulation, and there were quite logical reasons for this. First of all there is a rare inherited disease (called *familial hypercholesterolaemia* – FHC for short) in which blood cholesterol levels are *very* high and there is a corresponding high and early death rate from clotting diseases. FHC, which is a fairly rare condition, needs prompt and constant cholesterol-lowering treatment. But it was also noted that there was a common association between raised blood cholesterol in otherwise normal people (not suffering from FHC) and a tendency towards blood-clotting diseases in certain population groups. Finally, it was noted that so-called atheromatous disease (in which a cholesterol-based patch becomes deposited in the walls of blood vessels, with an increase in blood clotting) tends to occur in folk who also had a raised blood cholesterol. All in all, this added up to the medical conclusion (which also filtered through to the media and thus to the general public) that cholesterol was the 'bad guy' lurking behind all thrombotic disease, and that all we needed to do was to lower our blood cholesterol – by avoiding cholesterol-rich foods, and by taking cholesterol-lowering drugs – and then all would be well. This, it is becoming increasingly demonstrated, is probably a fallacy.

Now it is being realised just how very important was Dr Sinclair's hypothesis (see pages 52–3). Hugh Sinclair, while he was eating an Eskimo diet, found that his blood cholesterol did not change very much – and that the Eskimos who, like him, had blood that was disinclined to clot, also enjoyed pretty normal blood cholesterol levels.

Furthermore, it has been known for some time that cholesterol plays a *useful* function in the body. It helps transport fat throughout the body via the bloodstream. (In fact, it is so vital to our well-being that if there is not enough cholesterol in the blood, then the body manufactures some more!) It has also been shown recently that if you eat too much cholesterol then the body needs an increased intake of EFAs or essential fatty acids (see Glossary) to cope with it efficiently and safely. Perhaps this is the nub of the whole cholesterol story.

Most foodstuffs that are high in *non*-essential fatty acids are also high in cholesterol, and the combination of these two dietary events leads to raised blood cholesterol *and* a raised incidence of artery and thrombosis disorders. But this is more due to EFA starvation than high-cholesterol food. In other words, the ultimate deficiency in the diet in those with artery and blood-clotting problems is probably an inadequate essential fatty acid intake.

Good Health-Food Management

Health food therapy has only a little to offer once advanced pathological changes in arteries have occurred. But early *preventative* health-food action against artery disease can, however, make an enormous difference in terms of better health.

MARINE OILS AND ARTERY PROBLEMS

One of the most convincing health-food successes concerns the important part that marine oils can play as health foods in the prevention of artery disease. Marine oils, for a start, are unsaturated, and they have a high EFA (essential fatty acid) content: this stimulates the production of prostaglandins that tend to decrease the facility that the blood has to clot.

Some of these marine oils are produced from the flesh of fish (whole fish oil). Others are manufactured from fish liver, e.g., cod liver oil. The marine oil preparations known as MAXEPA and Pulse have been widely used in research in Britain and have found considerable favour.

ANTIOXIDANTS AND ARTERY PROBLEMS

The antioxidants – Vitamins A, C, E and beta-carotene, plus the micronutrient selenium – are the ultimate health-food frontline attack against the free radicals (see Glossary) that attack tissues in the body. Free radicals can easily damage the cells that line our blood vessels – particularly the arteries.

Once damaged, these can start to harden and develop arteriosclerosis.

Antioxidants also prevent fat-clogging plaques containing cholesterol from forming in the arteries. If these form, they can become foci for blood-clotting activity, and so a thrombus forms and then there is coronary or stroke illness. Really large-scale intervention trials recently, involving thousands of people, have proved that at least one antioxidant, Vitamin E, can reduce this morbidity and mortality significantly.

Vitamin C and selenium are also significant.

GOOD BUYS

★ *Gold Standard*
- Marine oils containing added Vitamin E (MAXEPA, PULSE)
- Selenium-ACE (WASSEN).

See also: **Ageing; Cardiac Problems; Glossary; Cod Liver Oil; Marine Oils; Selenium; Vitamins A, C and E.**

ARTHRITIS AND RHEUMATISM

YOU will know exactly what you mean when you complain about your arthritis and rheumatism. But patients find that doctors and rheumatologists are unhappy to deal with generalities like 'rheumatics'. Often they are at pains to point out that the whole subject of rheumatology really is complex because it encompasses a vast spectrum of widely differing diseases, and that it is only the various *symptoms* that seem to unite it. These symptoms include pain, disability and usually a degree of deformity as the years pass.

Because the *pathology* (the basic cause) that lies behind rheumatism and arthritis is so very various, an attempt is often made to divide the disease up into groups. In *degenerative* disease (e.g. hip osteoarthritis) the joints behave as if they are 'worn out'. But in *rheumatoid* disease the joints behave as though they are 'inflamed' long before they degenerate. This, of course, only begins to describe the masses of diseases commonly called arthritis and rheumatism. A whole host of other 'rheumaticky' diseases exist: for example, osteoporosis, juvenile arthritis and soft tissue rheumatism (myalgia and fibrositis).

Orthodox Medical Management

This is as various, understandably, as the pathology. Naturally it centres on relieving pain, and alleviating the disability and deformity. The classical management of arthritis and rheumatism – drugs, physiotherapy, surgery, rehabilitation – often succeeds, but all too often it does not. One of the major snags in the medical management of rheumatism is a lack of any very useful *prognostic* information about any individual case of rheumatism which would allow one form of treatment to be compared to another.

In other words, there is no blood test – or any other test – that can tell the doctor that a patient is going to be, say, severely crippled by their rheumatism in a few years, or that he or she will probably jog along with not too much degeneration for the best part of a lifetime. If cases of 'bad' rheumatism and arthritis could only be spotted early, then it might be possible to make better use of some of the very powerful (if potentially dangerous) drugs in our possession early on in therapy with a view to tackling the disease at an early stage.

Usually all rheumatism and arthritis is treated with pain-killing and anti-inflammatory drugs. Later, if the disease seems not to be responding, then more potent anti-rheumatic drugs and/or surgery are considered. Only comparatively recently has the concept of health-food nutritional supplementation been considered at all as an adjunct to rheumatism management. Often such remedies are sought out when medical treatment fails. There is a case for much earlier use of nutritional supplement when symptoms are milder.

Good Health-Food Management

There appear to be two major principles that operate in this field: improvements brought about mainly as a result of prostaglandin manipulation; or improvement brought about by antioxidant therapy.

PROSTAGLANDINS AND ARTHRITIS

Prostaglandins (see Glossary) are locally-acting tissue hormones, and they require the essential fatty acids found in marine and plant oils. The fact that cod liver oil takers quite often find that their rheumatic symptoms are ameliorated now seems to be accepted by many medical authorities. That this may come about as a result of prostaglandin action seems to be highly likely.

Experimental controlled supplementation using MAXEPA, marine and other unsaturated oil products have shown that many rheumatic symptoms improve when patients are taking the supplement capsules, while no improvement occurs in patients taking placebo capsules. More important, perhaps, on cessation of the supplement rheumatic symptomatology tends to recur. Other studies suggest that Omega 3 fatty acids, in products such as MAXEPA, are more effective as an anti-rheumatic than Omega 6 fatty acids − evening primrose oil, for instance. (See page 186.)

Much of the published work in this field is 'uncontrolled' in terms of medical science, but convincing. Dr Donald Rudin in his book, *The Omega 3 Phenomenon* (Sidgwick & Jackson, 1987), analysed a group of 44 patients, 45 per cent of whom had osteoarthritis or soft tissue rheumatism. Some 50 per cent had rheumatoid arthritis. Nearly all of these patients experienced a remission of their arthritis while they took an Omega 3-rich diet. (In this study, linseed was the oil used.)

ANTIOXIDANTS AND ARTHRITIS AND RHEUMATISM

There is an increasing wealth of evidence stemming from those who study the natural history of diseases that free radicals are

---

EFA AND OMEGA

The name Omega plus a number refers to the varying positions of double bonds between carbon atoms in fat molecules. Omega 3 oils are more polyunsaturated than Omega 6 oils, and some agree that they are better because of this.

Marine oils and linseed oil are rich in Omega 3 EFAs (Essential fatty Acids, see Glossary); evening primrose oil is rich in Omega 6 EFAs.

	Omega 3 (%)	Omega 6 (%)
Linseed oil	60	20
Fish oil	30	20

---

associated with many of the so-called degenerative diseases (cancer, cardiovascular disease, rheumatism and cataract) and that a low dietary intake of the antioxidants (selenium, Vitamins A, C and E) is provocative in rheumatism.

In rather the same way as the benefits of cod liver oil were 'discovered' – in a wealth of spontaneous testimonials from the general public – the effects of antioxidant therapy in rheumatology were first disclosed by news from patients' self-support groups rather than from a medical trial.

It was members of the Arthritic Association, in a trial reported in the magazine *Here's Health* (see Selenium), who first showed how much Selenium-ACE (selenium plus Vitamins A, C and E) helped. This small trial may stimulate further interest in the use of antioxidants in the long-term prevention and management of rheumatic disease.

COPPER AND ARTHRITIS AND RHEUMATISM

A Danish study and two US studies (see Copper) suggested that injections of the micronutrient were safe and effective in the control of rheumatic disease. That copper is considered a 'cure' by sufferers is exhibited by the number of copper bracelets worn; the medical profession remains to be convinced.

GOOD BUYS

★ *Gold standard*
- Marine oil products and linseed oil ● Omega 3 EFAs.

Useful
- An antioxidant supplement containing selenium and the Vitamins A, C and E, e.g. Selenium-ACE (WASSEN).

Worth Trying
- Seemingly less effective, mussel products (e.g. Seatone products from HEALTHCRAFTS, a relatively expensive way of getting Omega 3 EFAs).

See also: **Glossary; Osteoporosis; Cod Liver Oil; Copper; Evening Primrose Oil; Marine Oil; Plant Oils; Selenium; Vitamins A, C and E.**

BALDING, SCALP AND HAIR PROBLEMS

THE extent to which nutritional factors are involved in hair and scalp health is controversial. Hair is basically a 'dead' structure, like nails. Whether your hair looks healthy or not depends to a large extent on the sheen imparted to the hair shafts by the sebaceous glands that lubricate the hair, together with the presence or absence of scalp skin scaling debris – a natural process that has been christened dandruff.

But there are a few nutritional problems that damage hair at the *live* end, i.e. the hair root; the scalp skin is also influenced by good or poor nutrition.

Signs and Symptoms

Baldness occurs when hair loss persistently exceeds hair regeneration and growth. It is largely genetically programmed, and influenced very much by gender. Male-pattern baldness is a classic demonstration of this biological home truth. Some women can experience hair loss after childbirth or after giving up the Pill; many menopausal women find that their hair becomes much thinner. Cancer patients undergoing radiation or chemotherapy can lose their hair.

Many of the aspects relative to hair loss and the health of the scalp are poorly understood, particularly with reference to alopecia (sudden hair loss), in which psychological factors are very much involved. But embryology tells us that the skin and the central nervous system both develop from the same type of ectodermal cells in the very early days of life in the womb.

Orthodox Medical Management

In the case of balding, this is largely non-existent, other than hair transplantation. Steroid creams are often used in the treatment of alopecia. Some forms of dandruff require medical attention.

GOOD BUYS

As indicated opposite.

See also: **Pollen, Propolis and Royal Jelly; Iron; Marine Oils; Vitamins A, B and C; Zinc.**

GOOD HEALTH-FOOD MANAGEMENT OF HAIR PROBLEMS

Factor	*Therapy*
1. Prolonged protein lack (most commonly seen in long-stay institutionalised patients, but also in those who go on a protein-free diet)	High protein or amino acid diet (see Pollen, Propolis and Royal Jelly).
2. Chronic Vitamin A deficiency (hair loss complicated by excessive dandruff)	Vitamin A supplement.
3. Chronic Vitamin C deficiency (hair is misshapen, tangles easily, forms unusual patterns, scalp dry)	Daily small doses of Vitamin C.
4. Iron deficiency (often in anaemia, generally-distributed hair loss or alopecia)	Iron supplementation.
5. Zinc deficiency (hair loss associated with excessive scalp dryness)	Zinc supplementation.
6. Lacklustre hair and excessive dandruff	Marine oil supplementation. (Veterinarians make regular use of marine oils in the feeds of race horses and show horses, to improve the sheen on their coats.)

BED SORES

ALSO known as pressure sores, these start as an area of skin damage and, unless carefully treated, commonly develop into ulcers (lack of skin continuity). They are caused by excessive or constant pressure on parts of the skin and a consequent restriction of blood supply to the area. Bed sores are most common in those who are bedridden after illness or because of age. (They are a particular problem for the elderly who already have a poor skin blood supply, and diabetics.) Pressure sores are also common in hemiplegics and paraplegics, or those who are confined to a chair or wheelchair, for example, multiple sclerosis victims.

The most vulnerable points are where the bones lie near the skin – the buttocks and lower spine, the elbows, ankles and heels and particularly in those who are thin and have little fat to 'insulate' them from pressure. The less the patient moves or is moved, the more liable he or she is to develop the problem. The skin discolours, cracks and weeps, then forms the cavities of ulcers.

Orthodox Medical Management

Getting patients out of bed several times a day whenever possible, and the frequent turning of patients in bed, about once every 2 hours, physiotherapy and massage are the aims of good management. The provision of special mattresses, rings, cushions, Spenco 'ripple' beds and water beds are also a great boon. (These latter distribute the weight more evenly than conventional mattresses.)

Good nutritional management is important as well. This involves a good mixed diet which provides enough food to prevent excessive weight loss. Frequent weight checks are important.

Good Health-Food Management

VITAMIN C AND BED SORES

A study reported in the *British Journal of Nutrition* 20 years ago demonstrated that 23 per cent of a large group of paraplegics suffering from pressure sores had low levels of Vitamin C in their white blood corpuscles. (Testing for nutrients in blood corpuscles often gives more realistic evidence of vitamin status than when 'whole' blood is used.) Two years later a double blind study showed that areas of pressure-sore ulceration decreased in size by an average of 84 per cent when patients were given 500mg of Vitamin C twice daily for one month.

ZINC AND BED SORES

Zinc ointment has been used for centuries on wounds of all kinds, but oral zinc has been shown, in many studies, to be particularly effective in the healing of ulcers (see page 295).

GOOD BUYS

★ *Gold Standard*
• Both zinc and Vitamin C preparations would seem to be eligible for Gold Standard consideration in cases of venous and trophic ulceration.

Regular provision of Vitamin C supplement is mandatory because very little Vitamin C is stored in the body. Some nutritionists believe that once Vitamin C is given as a supplement it should be continued indefinitely.

See also: **Diabetes; Multiple Sclerosis; Varicose Veins, Ulcers and Haemorrhoids; Vitamin C; Zinc.**

BIRTH DEFECTS

NEURAL-TUBE defect or spina bifida (literally, divided spine) is one of the more common birth defects throughout the world. In spina bifida part of one or more vertebrae in a baby's spine fails to develop properly. This can leave the spinal cord exposed. It can occur anywhere in the backbone, but most commonly in the lower part of the back. The severity of the disability depends on how much of the spinal cord remains unprotected because of the defect. In the UK 40 babies in every 100,000 born have a spina bifida defect, and the rate is highest in the babies of relatively young or relatively old mothers. Once a woman gives birth to a spina bifida baby she is ten times more likely to have a similarly affected baby in a subsequent pregnancy.

The basic developmental 'mistake' that results in a baby being born with spina bifida occurs very early on in pregnancy – within four weeks of conception. It is possible to detect the presence or absence of spina bifida by means of sophisticated ultrasound scanning or biochemical tests very early on in pregnancy. This means that high-risk mothers, those who have already had a spina bifida baby, can (if they wish) opt for a pregnancy termination if tests confirm that the current baby is suffering from spina bifida.

Orthodox Medical Management

The degree of physical disability in a spina bifida victim depends on the severity of the developmental defect. A very mild degree of spina bifida is labelled *spina bifida occulta,* in which a small tuft of hair is sited over a very minor degree of defective spinal development and the child is in every other way normal. At the other end of the scale is a very severe form of the disability known as *myelocele.* Such a child is severely handicapped; the legs are paralysed, and there is loss of feeling and function below the level in the spine where the defect occurs. There are also bladder and bowel problems, and sometimes associated brain abnormalities, for instance hydrocephalus, develop.

Such a heavily handicapped child has to face up to neonatal surgery (to attempt to 'close' the defect), catheterisation to help with urinary problems, and a life subsequently dominated by wheelchairs, physiotherapy, intermittent hospitalisation and, if he or she survives, special schools and walking aids.

Good Health-Food Management

It has long been suspected that diet plays a role in preventing spina bifida defects, and the possibility that a vitamin of the B group, folate or folic acid, might be involved was first raised over a quarter of a century ago (in 1964). But it was not until the early 1980s that intervention studies were published which suggested that folate or other vitamin supplementation to the diet of women *very early on in their pregnancy* was followed by a reduced number of spina bifida babies being born.

Unfortunately, these early trials were not planned or carried out in such a way that they won the unqualified approval of the whole medical and nutritional establishment. (This seems to happen quite frequently in the world of nutrition.) Indeed, it was argued that the lower incidence of spina bifida in the folate takers was merely because these women were females coming from a selected, health-conscious fraction of the community who ate rather well, or at least better than did their less fortunate sisters.

However, in 1991 a prolonged international, double blind randomised trial, involving 33 centres (17 in the UK and 16 in six other countries) was published. Women who were planning to risk another pregnancy after once giving birth to a spina bifida baby were eligible for the study. These women were split into four groups, as shown in the table below.

Group	Folate	Other Vitamins
A	Yes	No
B	Yes	Yes
C	No	No
D	No	Yes

This trial was terminated early because it was obvious that results obtained were sufficiently conclusive, and to continue the 'No' groups put mothers at spina bifida risk. It was demonstrated that folate had a 72 per cent protective effect on spina bifida outcome. (A significant protective effect was demonstrated in the other vitamin groups tested as well.) A firm conclusion was reached by the MRC Study Group who carried out this mammoth trial, that it can be confidently recommended that folate supplementation *starting before pregnancy* has a very significant protective effect as far as spina bifida is concerned.

The supplements used in the study were prepared and packaged by Boots in two-week calendar 'blister' packs in a daily dosage of 4mg of folate. Pregnavite Forte F (Goldshield Pharmaceuticals), seems similarly protective and has been used in UK antenatal clincs for some time now.

Many physicians are now convinced that all women at risk of pregnancy should take a folate supplement, and those who decide our health policy are at the moment trying to make up their minds as to whether fortifying food with folate, or taking a health-food supplement, is the best way to reduce the risks of having a spina bifida baby.

Although it is still imperfectly understood why folate is so important – is it diet? or is it partially environmental? – folate has emerged as a health food *par excellence*.

GOOD BUYS

★ *Gold Standard*
● Folate tablets, 4mg daily ● Pregnavite Forte F (GOLDSHIELD PHARMACEUTICALS) 1 tablet daily.

To be fully effective, tablets have to be taken at the time of conception. In practice this means daily dosage throughout a woman's fertile life unless efficient contraception or sexual abstinence is practised.

See also: **Vitamin B (Folate).**

CANCER

APART from spectacular and isolated successes in the management of certain cancers (for example, testicular cancer, some skin cancers and certain leukaemias) the orthodox medical control of cancer has, generally speaking, been rather disappointing to date. But it would be extremely foolish to turn to health foods or any other form of alternative medicine with a view to ignoring or changing good medical or surgical advice. Perhaps the greatest success in cancer control on a worldwide basis has been the knowledge that certain very common cancers (of the lung and skin) can be largely *prevented* by stopping smoking and by limiting exposure to high levels of sunlight on a long-term basis.

But a strong body of medical and scientific opinion claims that further gains in cancer survival could be brought about by means of dietary manipulation, and the National Academy of Sciences in the USA estimates that 60 per cent of women's cancers and 40 per cent of cancers in men are related to nutritional factors. The value of a low-fat, high-fibre diet, and the avoidance of large quantities of smoked or salt-cured foods, are advocated with this aim in view.

Large-scale studies (that have mostly involved the micro-nutrient selenium) have convincingly demonstrated that the blood levels of certain nutrients are lower in cancer victims than in healthy controls. A debate continues as to whether there is a *causal* relation, however, and missing, to date, are large-scale human studies linking nutritional supplementation with an improved prognosis once a cancer is established. But many workers believe both in a preventative and a therapeutic role for health supplements in the fight against cancer. A short appraisal of the present position follows. See also the Glossary for information on the antioxidants.

VITAMIN A AND LUNG CANCER

Vitamin A may be taken into the body either from fish liver

oils, offal and dairy produce, or as a vegetable precursor called beta-carotene (the orange-coloured ingredient of carrots and fruit, and dark green vegetables). This beta-carotene is transformed into Vitamin A and absorbed into the body in the intestine. This curious animal/vegetable substance is in an odd and inexplicable way related to death risks from lung cancer. Scientific papers have started to report that if there is a lower than normal beta-carotene level in the blood of a particular population group, then this group also has a higher than normal chance of dying of lung cancer. This finding was more or less shrugged off as an obscure haematological finding until something of a nutritional bombshell was dropped. The *Lancet* published in 1981 the results of a 19-year prospective study (see Glossary) of 1,954 patients which demonstrated that there was an inverse relationship between the *intake* of beta-carotene and the incidence of lung cancer. For some inexplicable reason, a high blood beta-carotene level seemed to reduce the likelihood of developing lung cancer. This lifted the whole problem out of the laboratory and into the greengrocery and health food market!

Five years later, in 1986, the *New England Journal of Medicine* published a study which compared levels of beta-carotene in the blood of lung cancer patients and matched controls of non-cancer patients. This again showed an inverse relationship between the level of beta-carotene in the blood and lung cancer. It has been quite rightly pointed out that all this means is that if you are suffering from lung cancer then this upsets your beta-carotene status. Advocates of the theory that there is a more positive dietary link would say that low beta-carotene levels in your blood makes cancer of the lung rather more likely to develop in you or me than in the people next door if they enjoy a high beta-carotene blood level. Thus belief is forged that anything you do to improve your blood beta-carotene levels improves your chances of escaping cancer of the lung.

VITAMINS A, C AND E AND LARYNX CANCER

Cancer of the larynx (voice box) is strongly linked with smoking and chronic high alcohol intake. But quite extensive studies published in reputable medical journals have demonstrated that where amounts of Vitamins A and C in the diet are low there is also an increased risk of this cancer developing. Many other studies have disclosed unexpected links between a deficiency of certain other vitamins (especially C and E) and cancer risk generally. The whole subject is excellently and scientifically reviewed in Dr Melvyn R. Werbach's important book, *Nutritional Influences on Illness* (Thirdline Press Inc., New Canaan, 1988). See also Antioxidants (Glossary).

FIBRE AND BOWEL CANCER

Cancer of the large bowel is the second most common cancer in the West, and there would appear to be undisputed links between its occurrence and diet. People who live in the country seem to be less affected by this particular cancer, probably due to their diet containing more fibre than that of the town-dweller. To cut down on risks of developing bowel cancer (and many others), it is advisable that fibre intake should be increased.

FOLATE AND CERVICAL CANCER

It has been noted that blood levels of folate, a member of the B vitamin complex, are low in cervical cancer patients. It has also been shown that the proliferation of pre-cancerous cells (cervical dysplasia) can be reduced by folate supplementation.

SELENIUM AND CANCER

With the increased interest in, and excitement about, antioxidant therapy, selenium has emerged from several trials and studies as a cancer preventative or prophylactic *par excellence*. Those who live in or near selenium-rich soil areas seem to be better protected against cancers developing; and those with good levels of blood selenium would appear to be less at risk too.

Good Buys

★ *Gold Standard*
- Selenium tentatively established.

Useful
- Beta-carotene products, e.g. Beta-carotene (QUEST)
- Fibre • Selenium/Vitamin C and E products, e.g. Selenium-ACE (WASSEN) • Folate products.

See also: **Ageing; Glossary; Fibre; Selenium; Vitamins A, B (folate), C and E.**

Candidiasis (Thrush)

ANY vaginal discharge needs to be investigated medically so that an accurate diagnosis can be established. One common type of vaginal discharge, a fungal infection called *candidiasis,* can be helped by good health food management.

Signs and Symptoms

The commonest symptom is vaginal itching. This can vary from the barely discernible to the totally intolerable, in which case vaginal soreness and burning, especially during and after intercourse, is experienced. Sometimes a vaginal discharge occurs and sometimes, too, there is soreness when urine is passed. The soreness can spread to adjacent skin areas.

In some cases candidiasis spreads to the vagina from the bowel. The basic cause in such cases is a yeast-like fungus called *Candida albicans.*

PREDISPOSING FACTORS

1. *Humidity:* poor clothes ventilation, too many clothes, nylon pants and tights, 'tropical' environment (real or induced).

2. *Hormone influences:* pre-menstrual, contraceptive pill, pregnancy, steroid drugs.

3. *General illness:* diabetes.

4. *Removal of natural control:* antibiotic treatments foster candidiasis.

5. *Lowered immunity:* severe anaemia, some malignancies, some drugs.

Orthodox Medical Management

There is a variety of medical treatments available in the form of pessaries, tablets, creams, medicated tampons and anti-fungal drugs. Predisposing factors should be eliminated as far as possible.

Good Health-Food Management

Yoghurt has been shown to be helpful in restoring the normal bacterial flora and fauna which allow the body to combat candidiasis. Eat it or apply it to the affected areas. Acidophilus preparations are similarly helpful.

GOOD BUYS

- Acidophilus Plus (QUEST) • Acidophilus Extra (LAMBERT'S)
- Acidophilus (NATURE'S OWN).

These are health foods containing a high concentration of 'friendly' bacteria which inhibit over-growth of *Candida* in the bowel and allow the vagina to resume its normal ecology.

CARDIAC PROBLEMS

WE in the UK have an unenviable cardiac health reputation. About half a million of us in England and Wales have a heart attack (myocardial infarct) in any given year. Up to half of those who do so die, usually without having seen a doctor, let alone being admitted to a hospital coronary care unit.

A search for better cardiac health has spread the medical message that heart attacks are associated with multi-factorial causes. Some of the factors involved (e.g. artery problems, high blood cholesterol and disturbances of blood pressure) have been extensively researched and acted upon. As a result the death rate from heart attack is decreasing, especially in the USA and in Australia and Europe. But in the UK this is happening more slowly. Where such improvements in mortality have occurred, these have been gained either as a result of a decrease in smoking and/or adoption of healthier lifestyles associated with changes in diet and in exercise patterns.

Basically the heart is a pump, and it is cardiac power-failure that produces most heart problems (although there is a wide spectrum of heart disease that exists outside this important concept, valvular and congenital diseases of the heart, for example). Power-failure in the heart usually comes about as a result of heart *muscle* failure, for the heart's muscle is the sole source of its power and force. Muscles need nutrients if they are to work efficiently, and these nutrients come in three main forms. First of all, there is oxygen, the prime nutrient of all our cells, including muscle cells. Second, there is a need for fuel (as glucose) which you might say is the heart's 'petrol'. The third class of nutrients essential to a hard-working and efficient heart are the essential minerals.

US cardiologist Dr W. Raab has made a name for himself as a tireless researcher into the whole field of cardiology, and he feels that the 'official' approach to much cardiac disease is often based on outdated concepts. Dr Raab caused a stir at a symposium on myocardiology a few years ago by claiming that in about half the deaths clinically attributed to myocardial infarction, coronary occlusion, coronary thrombosis (all synonyms for coronary thrombosis), *no* thrombi (clots) or vascular occlusion (blocked artery) can be found subsequently at autopsy at all! And he put forward the theory that it was changes in the heart muscle electro-chemistry that were really 'stopping the clock' in such cases.

According to Dr Raab's scenario of sudden death from a heart attack, a state of affairs develops, first of all, in which there is some impairment of heart muscle oxygenation, due to a degree of hardening of the arteries (see also page 179). This lowers the amount of oxygen that is permeating the heart muscle, and causes several effects, including a lowering of the heart muscle's store of essential minerals. Should a stress situation now occur, be it psychological or physical, suddenly the heart demands even more oxygen. In such circumstances the heart's action can lose its natural rhythm and start to beat in a disorderly and inefficient way. In some circumstances it can actually stop.

Apart from the serious sudden-death type of emergencies that Dr Raab has drawn attention to, there is a wide spectrum of cardiac upset which makes many people's lives a misery. These include what are called paroxysmal tachycardia attacks, a condition in which, for no known reason in most cases, the heart suddenly starts to race and frightening palpitations are experienced, often at night. Paroxysmal tachycardia patients may or may not have a degree of coronary artery disease.

Normally, our heart beats at between 60 and 90 beats a minute and, although we can feel it at the wrist or in our neck, we normally do not notice it. But if, under exertion or excitement, it increases to well above 100 beats per minute, palpitation is obvious.

The electrical circuitry of the heart is normally centred in a small collection of cells called the sino-atrial node, and this is surrounded by cells of the autonomic (automatic) nervous system. These are connected to the central nervous system and so when you are excited or frightened your brain communicates directly with your sino-atrial node and tells your heart to speed up – maybe you are going to be in for some action!

Orthodox Medical Management

This tends to be pharmacological on the whole, as in Artery Problems on page 179 – 80.

Good Health-Food Management

Health foods can be very useful in dealing with arterial heart disease (see also Artery Problems), but can do little in the case of heart failure. However, some health foods have been identified as being involved in better cardiac health, particularly the essential fatty acids and the antioxidants (see Glossary).

COD LIVER OIL AND CARDIAC PROBLEMS

All the marine oils, particularly cod liver oil, possess properties that decrease the blood's tendency to clot. This is, of course, vital in avoiding heart attacks through thrombosis.

GARLIC AND CARDIAC PROBLEMS

Recent studies of cardiac 'black spots' in the UK have come up with the suggestion that garlic – which has been extensively used in trials for other diseases such as hypertension – could be prophylactic.

MAGNESIUM AND CARDIAC PROBLEMS

Of the minerals essential for heart health, magnesium is well to the fore, having a stabilising effect on the heart's neuro-circuitry. If the organ becomes deficient in the mineral, any sudden excess of stress, whether psychological or physical, can make the heart palpitate, lose its rhythm or, in extreme cases, stop. These irregularities can occur after heart surgery, and again low-serum magnesium levels were found to be involved.

One of the baffling things about sudden death from heart disease has always been the protective effect, from the heart's point of view, of living in a hard-water area. Residents of hard-water areas in the USA, such as Omaha and Nebraska, as well as people living in London, all have a much better chance of not dying suddenly from heart attack than those who are soft-water drinkers, like residents of the soft-water cities of the south-eastern USA and people in the soft-water areas around Glasgow in Scotland. It is highly significant that hard water contains more magnesium than does soft water. Hard-water drinkers get a lot of their day-to-day magnesium from their tap water.

SELENIUM AND CARDIAC PROBLEMS

Because of its antioxidant properties, selenium can be particularly helpful in the heart problems that occur through artery disease. There is a high prevalence of coronary heart disease around Karelia, in Finland; the people there have a low selenium concentration in their blood, and there is a low selenium content in the soil. There is evidence that the authorities are trying to add selenium to their depleted soil so as to improve the selenium content of their grain in a natural way. But it looks as though this is a long and expensive process. Selenium supplementation would seem to be the more effective.

A severe selenium deficiency is related to the development of a form of heart muscle disease in children and animals.

GOOD BUYS

• Marine oil products • Garlic and garlic products • Magnesium products • Selenium-ACE (WASSEN).

See also: **Ageing; Artery Problems; Glossary; Hypertension; Cod Liver Oil; Garlic; Magnesium; Marine Oils; Selenium; Vitamins A, C and E.**

CARPAL TUNNEL SYNDROME

THIS disease, which is commonest in women between the ages of 40 and 60, also occurs in golfers of both sexes, and manifests itself in episodes of pain, tingling or aches of the muscles in the hand. These symptoms commonly wake the victims from sleep, or the pain may be present on waking. Shaking the hands or immersion in warm water often relieves the discomfort to start with, but if the condition becomes chronic the symptoms persist and some noticeable wasting and weakness of the small muscles of the thumb occurs.

The basic cause of the syndrome is unknown, but clearly the symptoms are caused by compression of nerves as they leave the arm and enter the hand. Similar conditions occur much less commonly elsewhere in the body and are referred to as 'nerve entrapment syndromes' by orthopaedic surgeons.

Orthodox Medical Management

Most of the common remedies for pain relief are ineffective, but the condition is usually cured by either steroid injections into the wrist or by a surgical operation to divide the fibrous band that normally keeps tendons, blood vessels and nerves snugly in position over the wrist joint.

Good Health-Food Management

This can hardly be said to be highly satisfactory, and conventional (orthopaedic) treatment is most effective. Some investigators have, however, advocated the use of high doses of pyridoxine (Vitamin B$_6$), but it has been demonstrated that such a dosage continued over several months (100mg daily) can itself be associated with neuritis. The *Lancet* has reported negative results after such high-dosage B$_6$ therapy, and the only cases in which B$_6$ seemed to reduce symptoms were those in which a B$_6$ deficiency was found. This is rare in practice.

Nevertheless, if you are wary of surgery, you could take

pyridoxine in daily doses of up to 100mg, providing no signs of neuritis (pins and needles sensations in limbs) complicate therapy.

GOOD BUYS

● Pyridoxine, 50mg tablets ● Time Release Vitamin B complex (HEALTHCRAFTS).

See also: **Vitamin B₆.**

CATARACT

CATARACT is loss of transparency of the crystalline lens of the eye, and is due to ageing changes which take place in the protein fibres of the lens. (This is not unlike what happens to the white of an egg when you boil it.) For reasons that we do not understand, opacification occurs in most people's eye lens, to some extent, once they pass the age of 65, although it can of course occur much earlier.

Signs and Symptoms

Cataract usually appears in both eyes. The symptoms are of a slowly progressive blurring of vision, often made worse in high light intensities. Sometimes colour perception is altered, too – blues are dulled, reds, yellows and oranges are accentuated. Often the blurring of vision makes night driving unsafe as a cataract matures and becomes more dense.

Orthodox Medical Management

It is extraordinarily easy to restore the lost vision of advanced cataract by means of a simple operation, the prototype of which was performed by the ancients. Eventually, when doctors invented spectacles, a thick cataract spectacle lens could restore a greater degree of vision after cataract surgery. Today, sophisticated cataract surgery makes use of lens implants, and very effective and routine cataract operations form a larger part of ophthalmological practice throughout the world.

Good Health-Food Management

As recently as 1985 an eminent ophthalmic surgeon with a world-wide reputation could state categorically that 'There is no known method of delaying the process of cataract or of clearing the opacities, short of removing the cataractous lens, although bogus therapies abound.'

ANTIOXIDANTS AND CATARACT

Recent work, hailing mostly from the USA and Canada, is however questioning at least the first part of that surgical diktat, and an increasing wealth of information states that dietary factors seem to impinge rather importantly on cataract prevention. Preliminary work along these lines was presented at an international conference on Antioxidant Vitamins and Beta-Carotene in Disease Prevention held in London in 1989.

Professor Paul Jacques, of the Human Nutrition Center for Aging at Tufts University, Boston, USA, compared the blood levels and dietary intake of the antioxidant Vitamins E, C and beta-carotene in a study of 112 of his patients, 77 of whom had one or more cataracts and compared them with 35 cataract-free patients. It was discovered that people with low blood levels of Vitamin C had eleven times the risk of developing cataract and those with low levels of beta-carotene had seven times the risk of cataract. This convinced him that a case for health-food supplementation with a view to cataract prevention should be considered.

A Canadian study from the University of Western Ontario has examined the cataract problem from a different viewpoint – the self-reported use of vitamin supplements in

175 patients. The study compared this group with 175 cataract-free patients. A significantly greater use of Vitamins E and C was found in the cataract-free group. The overall reduction rate in cataract risk in supplement takers was around 30 per cent. A very large prospective trial in the USA which involved over 5,000 women has shown very recently (1992) that both Vitamin C and carotenoids decrease the risk of cataract. (Carotenoids are substances derived from carrots, such as beta-carotene.) A randomised controlled trial is awaited, but it would seem to be substantially suggested that if vitamin supplementation in those over the age of 60 is maintained, then expensive and possibly traumatic surgery for cataract removal in the over-65 age groups could be substantially reduced.

A daily dose of a supplement containing RNIs of beta-carotene and Vitamins E and C would seem to be indicated. To date no combination product designed to cater for this important group seems to be marketed. Several beta-carotene products are available in health-food outlets in 5 – 15mg doses. Price will dictate the best buy.

GOOD BUYS

● Multi-vitamin preparations (beta-carotene, Vitamins E and C) ● Beta-carotene capsules (QUEST) ● Any multi-vitamin product containing beta-carotene is a good buy.

See also: **Ageing; Glossary; Vitamin A, C and E.**

COLDS

IT has been estimated that in the USA $1 billion is spent every year on cold remedies. In the UK there is a smaller but active over-the-counter market in cold remedies designed to make the unpleasant symptoms easier to bear for the week or so, two or three times a year, during which most of us have to put up with a cold.

Colds are caught by breathing in virus-containing droplets that have been coughed or sneezed into the atmosphere by a cold sufferer. Or perhaps by rubbing eyes or nose with fingers that have picked up a virus through hand-to-hand contact with a cold sufferer, or by the handling of infected handkerchiefs or towels.

Signs and Symptoms

Colds differ greatly in their signs and symptoms. Bad colds are often indistinguishable from influenza or hayfever in the summer months.

Orthodox Medical Management

Physicians point out that there are 200 or so viruses that are associated with the production of the symptoms of the common cold, and that no convincing trials have indicated any medication which will either prevent, shorten or cure colds.

The medications most commonly used are aspirin and paracetamol-containing preparations which combat the painful side of cold symptomatology (headache, muscular aches and pains, sore throat and chest), or by decongestants which temporarily shrink down swollen mucous membranes in the nose and allow for easier breathing. Various cough mixtures make coughs less painful and frequent. All such remedies have potential side effects – gastric irritation, 'rebound' symptomatology in the case of decongestants, and drowsiness which may be hazardous to those involved in driving or the operation of machinery. These side effects are always a potential danger to cough mixture or linctus takers. (Often certain cold preparations are best taken at night time to minimise the effect of such complications.) Very simple preparations – for example, menthol and eucalyptus pastilles – help make cold symptoms less worrying and avoid troublesome side effects.

Good Health-Food Management

In the face of such a tremendous potential market it is perhaps surprising that health food manufacturers have not been able to make a more satisfactory contribution to the great and prolonged fight for an effective remedy. Here and there, however, claims have been made for particular products.

VITAMIN C AND COLDS

The well-remembered Linus Pauling who, as a Nobel Prize-winning scientist, spent much of his later years advocating megadoses of Vitamin C as a cold prophylactic and cure, was probably responsible for hundreds of thousands of cold sufferers swallowing 1g of Vitamin C once, twice or thrice to abort a cold, or to make its earliest stages less troublesome. Regrettably no Gold Standard clinical trial ever proved or disproved this mega Vitamin C therapy for colds, and today there are fewer advocates.

HOMOEOPATHIC PRODUCTS AND COLDS

Dr Marjory Blackie, for many years the Queen's homoeopathic physician, used to tell her students at the Royal Homoeopathic Hospital that both her own and presumably her patron's favourite remedy for the common cold was homoeopathic *Allium* (onion). This is a remedy which incidentally demonstrates rather well the homoeopathic credo of *similia similibus curantur* (like cures like), in which the administration of minute amounts of a substance which in larger quantities will produce the symptoms of a disease is a potential cure of the bothersome disease. Anyone who peels and chops an onion will verify this particular homoeopathic axiom in action.

ZINC AND COLDS

Perhaps the most interesting recent claim for a health food remedy for colds comes from an organic chemistry professor whose work won him an endowed lectureship and silver medal from the Royal Society of Chemistry. Professor Derek Bryce-Smith's book, *The Zinc Solution* is possibly the most authoritative popular source on the biomedicine of zinc.

One very important proviso when considering any health food in any context is, of course, that the substance under consideration actually works, is non-toxic in recommended doses and is supported by substantial clinical trials. Unfortunately, clinical trials on something as variable and ill-defined as the common cold have baffled and confused even the very élite of the medico-scientific community, and recently the UK Government's Common Cold Research Unit at Salisbury was finally closed. An appraisal of its work leads me to the conclusion that not a lot was learned from the mass of careful and dedicated work carried out by its scientific personnel.

As far as zinc therapy is concerned, there is little to indicate that it was seriously considered at Salisbury. Nevertheless, Professor Derek Bryce-Smith refers us to several persuasive studies which would seem to indicate that zinc can help prevent colds, and shorten their duration (see Zinc).

IRON AND COLDS

Another, but largely anecdotal, cold cure crops up in the interesting therapeutic area of medical practice where so-called tonics and health foods meet. There is a condition well known to the carers of young children, but largely overlooked by the medical profession, in which toddlers suffer from cold after cold (on average, up to ten times a year). It is difficult in retrospect to find out whether it was a doctor, a mother or a pharmacist who first thought of prescribing an iron tonic – marketed as *Minadex* – for such children.

Minadex is considered by most doctors to be something of a therapeutic hotch-potch. It is an orange-flavoured syrup containing Vitamins A and D, iron, glycophosphates and micronutrient doses of manganese and copper. In short, Minadex is the sort of 'medicine' that would make the average scientific doctor smile quietly, and do his best to change the subject.

Curiously, perhaps (and for years Minadex was a medicine prescribable under the NHS), Minadex gained an enviable reputation with the mothers who dosed their children with it for recurrent and troublesome colds. Perhaps one day someone will organise a scientific trial that could result in deciding whether Minadex or Nature cures the recurrent cold syndrome in toddlers.

It is more than possible that small children, especially poor and faddy eaters, could have immune systems less than fully supported by certain protective nutrients and that good, old-fashioned Minadex very cleverly repairs that defect in a quite straightforward, if unsuspected, way.

SELENIUM AND COLDS

That the immune system is highly sensitive to dietary manipulation and deprivation has very recently been demonstrated in a study carried out in Belgium and reported upon in a much-respected US nutritional journal (see Selenium). This was a rather specialised study that sought out and observed one well-recognised scientific indication of a person's immune status. This is the response that our white blood corpuscles make to an immunological challenge, in this case an allergic challenge to a plant mitogen. (It must be explained that a delayed immunological response can, by means of this rather complicated incursion into the body's biochemistry, be measured scientifically.) The trial seemed to confirm that selenium can be immunostimulatory in elderly people, which could point the way towards the micronutrient being used as a prophylactic as far as colds and other infections are concerned.

GOOD BUYS

A bad cold can be made less traumatic by the administration of any of the popular cold remedies available in pharmacies and elsewhere. There is an advantage in buying from a pharmacy because a good pharmacist will indicate contraindications and side effects of certain preparations.

• Minadex is worth trying for children • Convinced homoeopaths may wish to try Allium 30, two tablets dissolved under the tongue, thrice daily • Zinc therapy is best taken in lozenge form for sore throat symptoms, or as tablets, e.g. Vitamin C + Zinc (HEALTHCRAFTS), for more general cold symptoms • Selenium therapy (Selenium-ACE – WASSEN) would seem particularly worthwhile for those who live institutionally or for grandparents who catch grandchildren's colds on a regular basis.

See also: **Allergy; Hayfever; Immunodepression; Homoeopathic Products; Iron; Selenium; Vitamin C; Zinc.**

CONSTIPATION

CONSTIPATION is difficult to define, and one person's constipation may be another's normal bowel habit. It is important, however, to try to decide what exactly *is* a normal bowel habit, because a change of bowel habit can sometimes indicate the need for special bowel investigation.

Many people commonly experience an episode of constipation if their everyday mode of life undergoes a change, for example going away on holiday or into hospital. Given a little time in the changed environment, the bowel habit usually reasserts itself. But it is at this stage that many resort to unwise constipation medication. This may result in a prompt and satisfactory end to the initial episode of constipation, but could be followed by a further secondary constipation and therefore more laxatives. Sometimes this second treatment works less effectively, the laxative dose is increased, or stronger laxatives are used. All too often such a stop-go routine develops into a condition known as laxative habituation. In other words, the bowel becomes hooked on a laxative to keep it regular.

Signs and Symptoms

A good working definition of constipation is the infrequent and uncomfortable passage of hard stools. Infrequent in this context means fewer than three times a week. Such a definition must be further qualified because some people open their bowels three times a day and others only once a week or so, and, if this is unaccompanied by any problem, it can be considered normal for them. If there is some difficulty or discomfort involved in the passage of the stools, however, then this could be constipation.

Orthodox Medical Management

Usually doctors tend to follow the following therapeutic sequence in the management of constipation.

Stage 1: Bulking agents (bran, isphagula, stercolia, methylcellulose).

Stage 2: Motion-softening preparations used especially in potentially painful conditions (liquid paraffin, docusate sodium).

Stage 3: Osmotic laxatives (magnesium salts, lactitol, lactulose).

Stage 4: Stimulant laxatives (senna preparations, bisacodyl, phenolphthalein).

Doctors tend to avoid Stage 4 laxatives if possible because of risks of laxative habituation. Senna preparations are relatively free from this complication, and are gentler in action than other Stage 4 laxatives.

Good Health-Food Management

It is health-food products rather than medical research that have brought about major improvements in constipation management over the last few decades, and fibre has become the Gold Standard therapy.

However, it is important to bear in mind when increasing your daily fibre intake that you do it very slowly and gradually over weeks rather than days. Always be sure to increase fluid consumption as part of the routine as well. Unless this is remembered, due to the quicker bowel transit times that follow increasing fibre intake, intestinal gas pains and discomfort become a nuisance.

For the bowel is a very sensitive neuromuscular organ, and many built-in reflex functions are involved in symptom-free bowel transit and movement. One such reflex is the gastrocolic reflex in which distension of the stomach by food (or air) stimulates the colon – the storage organ where the body 'parks' food residues and absorbs water from them, until they reach the last part of the bowel (the rectum) from which the faeces are eliminated. The presence of bulky, fibre-rich stools in the upper bowel can speed up the whole transit system excessively, and if this acceleration is too rapid, undigested carbohydrate tends to undergo an internal fermentation process producing masses of (mostly methane) gas. This is harmless but can be uncomfortable or embarrassing when the elimination of excessive flatus (bowel gas) becomes necessary. Recurrent colicky bowel pain is often an indication that too much fibre is being taken.

If foods are the means by which an individual is trying to re-educate the bowel, then too much of the fibre rich foods known to produce intestinal 'wind' (beans, cauliflower, sprouts, broccoli) are best avoided. Finally, if a sensible exercise schedule can be adhered to, this helps enormously in the bowel re-education process for fibre takers.

FIBRE AND CONSTIPATION

When using 100 per cent cereal bran as an increased fibre

source to aid symptom-free and regular bowel functioning, do so gradually. Start by taking a heaped teaspoon of bran per day for three days. This can be taken in any (uncooked) way, adding it to fruit purées or yoghurt, say. After those three days, and for the next three days, increase the daily bran dose by a heaped teaspoonful. For a further three days, take three heaped teaspoonfuls of bran. Always take an extra 300ml (½ pint) fluid for each spoonful of bran. Once a regular easy bowel movement daily is accomplished without gas problems, stay with the extra fibre intake regimen indefinitely.

If constipation does not respond to this routine, consult a physician.

GOOD BUYS

Many of the medical-management remedies are available in pharmacists and health food shops – especially senna preparations, such as Senokot and senna tablets.

★ *Gold Standard*
• Bran is the Gold Standard therapy.

See also: **Fibre; Herbalist Products.**

CROHN'S DISEASE AND ULCERATIVE COLITIS

Ulcerative colitis, and a condition known as Crohn's Disease, are common but little-discussed problems. Doctors refer to both conditions as *non-specific inflammatory bowel disease,* which really means that something or other is making parts of the bowel appear reddened and inflamed (when viewed through a surgical instrument or during an operation), and nobody is too sure what the actual cause of the inflammation is! To some extent the part of the bowel that is inflamed influences the diagnosis. Crohn's Disease can affect any part of the gastro-intestinal tract, while ulcerative colitis affects only the large bowel. It is important for doctors to get the right diagnostic labels, as the medical treatment and health-food management of each condition are rather different. Special tests and investigations usually clinch the diagnosis.

A lot of people suffer from non-specific inflammatory bowel disease. Both ulcerative colitis and Crohn's Disease can occur at any age, but the peak incidence is between 20 and 40 years and both sexes are equally affected. Crohn's Disease affects about 40 per 100,000 people in the UK, while ulcerative colitis about 80 per 100,000 people. Both conditions have a worldwide distribution, and the condition is less common in non-white races and commonest in Jews. Both diseases show a puzzling geographical and family clustering that nobody has ever explained satisfactorily.

Signs and Symptoms

The symptoms of ulcerative colitis include frequent diarrhoea (with the passage of blood and mucus) and recurrent abdominal pain accompanied by general malaise, lethargy and loss of appetite. Sufferers are often reluctant to discuss their problems even with their doctors and families, and many have to face up to a lifetime of symptomatology not always alleviated by medical and sometimes surgical treatment.

Crohn's Disease is also known as ileitis, because the inflammation most commonly affects the ileum, the lower part of the small bowel. The bowel can become swollen through inflammation or ulceration, and the passage of faeces can be obstructed. Otherwise, many symptoms are as for ulcerative colitis.

Orthodox Medical Management

Both medical and surgical treatment have an enormous amount to contribute to effective management of both ulcerative colitis and Crohn's Disease – long-term antibiotic and steroid treatment, excision of diseased bowel – although many victims often explore fringe therapy and alternative medicine to ease their suffering. Fortunately, in Britain there is an efficient patients' association in the form of the National Association for Colitis and Crohn's Disease (at 98a London Road, St Albans, Herts AL1 1NX), and in other countries similar self-help organisations are evolving.

Good Health-Food Management

To a large extent this involves dietary manipulation. Some victims discover for themselves that certain foods upset them. Diets that are high in refined carbohydrates – sugary and sweet foods – are commonly believed to be bad for ulcerative colitis, but victims often react in a highly idiosyncratic way to foods.

VITAMINS A AND D IN ULCERATIVE COLITIS

In ulcerative colitis victims the oil-soluble Vitamins A and D together with calcium, magnesium and zinc have been reported to play a useful therapeutic role, although evidence in this matter is not strong. On a long-term basis it would seem that a multi-mineral/vitamin supplement can only improve the lot of the victim of non-specific inflammatory bowel disease.

217

FIBRE AND CROHN'S DISEASE

A fibre-rich diet has been shown to significantly reduce both the number and time-stay of patients admitted to hospital with Crohn's Disease.

GOOD BUYS

• These include vitamin and fibre products. It is important to avoid any tendency of fibre to produce intestinal flatulence and, although this is highly subjective, Linusit Gold (FINKS), Fibre Mix (JUVELA) and Rite-Diet (NUTRITIA) often find favour • Good buys in the multivitamin/mineral field would include Genesis (WASSEN) or multiple minerals, especially magnesium or zinc, and Vitamins B, A and D (QUEST).

See also: **Fibre; Vitamins A and D.**

DEPRESSION

THERE is an important difference between feeling depressed, which we all experience from time to time, and the psychiatric illness known as depression which, although very common, is not part of everyone's experience of life.

Signs and Symptoms

True depression is characterised by an abnormal lowering of mood, with sadness, melancholy and emotional dejection manifest. There is also what is called psychomotor retardation, in which all physical activity is severely curtailed. In most cases, a depression of body functions including appetite, libido, and an ability to sleep normally are experienced by the severely depressed person.

NUTRITIONAL FACTORS AND DEPRESSION

Nutrient	Evidence
Biotin (B group vitamin)	A small group of patients on a biotin-deficient diet became depressed – the condition was relieved by supplementation.
Folate (B group vitamin)	Depressed patients were found to have low blood folate levels. Depressed patients being treated with Lithium improved if given folate.
Pyridoxine (Vitamin B$_6$) (see page 126 re overdosage)	If blood pyridoxine is lowered (as it may be in 'contraceptive pill depression'), then this depression improved with supplementation. A placebo-controlled study has confirmed this.
Vitamin C	Over 10 per cent of 465 hospitalised psychiatric patients in the UK study were shown to be borderline Vitamin C-deficient. Vitamin C taken daily reduced the level of depression.

Orthodox Medical Management

Safe and proper management of depressive illness is purely a medical matter, and health-food products have only a small place in its alleviation. There are, however, some interesting correlations between depression and certain dietary deficiencies, and because depressed patients often have poor appetites these are worthwhile bearing in mind. In other words, we want to break any vicious circle which states 'My appetite and desire to eat is poor – I eat only poorly and under duress – I become depleted of vital nutrients – Because of this I am further depressed.'

GOOD BUYS

There is no Gold Standard product, but sensible consensus would seem to be that when long-term depression or other chronic psychiatric condition is associated with institutional-isation, or withdrawal from everyday living, then health-food supplementation with minerals and vitamins should be carefully considered.

• Any Vitamin B_6 (pyridoxine) product   • Any high-potency Vitamin C product   • Strezz B-Vite (HEALTHCRAFTS), which contains pyridoxine, biotin and folate in safe doses.

See also: **Tension and Stress; Vitamins B (Biotin, Folate and B_6) and C.**

DIABETES

DIABETES affects, in its various forms, some 30 million people world-wide. It is basically a metabolic abnormality that is characterised by an increased amount of sugar circulating in the blood, brought about by an abnormality of insulin production by the body. These days doctors talk about Type I (insulin-dependent) or Type II (non-insulin-dependent) diabetes (often called late-onset diabetes), which is sensible as they are really quite different diseases.

Orthodox Medical Management

This is primarily a matter for your doctor, and each diabetic needs individually-tailored treatment worked out by specialists with knowledge and expertise in diabetic management. This medical management always involves specialised dietary advice. As well as insulin, various drugs are prescribed as part of efficient diabetic *control*, for there is as yet no cure for diabetes.

Good Health-Food Management

Considerable interest has been shown in the role that certain vitamins, minerals and other nutrients may play in the management of diabetes, and particularly in the control of the secondary symptoms that arise from metabolic injury to the diabetic's arteries and nervous system. The antioxidant nutrients and minerals together with the B complex vitamins and GLA (gamma linolenic acid), have all been studied by various research groups, but with equivocal results. Vitamin E is considered to be so likely to favourably alter insulin requirements that one study advised all diabetics who added it to their diet to check with their physician in case they needed to *reduce* their insulin requirements.

DIABETES

Type I	Type II
	(sometimes called late–onset diabetes)
Younger	Older
Lean	Overweight
30 – 50 per cent concordance in identical twins	90 per cent concordance in identical twins
Insulin deficiency	Partial insulin deficiency and insulin resistance
Always need insulin	Sometimes need insulin
Signs and symptoms may include loss of weight, frequent infections, attacks of disturbed consciousness, slow-to-heal ulcers or other complications of diabetes (artery disease, cataract, coma attacks).	Signs and symptoms may be minimal other than obesity. Later complications of Type I diabetes develop if control is poor.

FIBRE AND DIABETES

Many studies have shown the efficacy of adding fibre to diabetic diets. Diabetics may even be able to thus *decrease* their intake of insulin, but only on the advice of their doctor.

POTASSIUM AND DIABETES

Potassium is important to diabetics, because sufficient dietary potassium is needed for the proper use of sugars.

GOOD BUYS

All diabetics who consider taking advantage of dietary supplementation with vitamins and minerals should consult their physician. If fibre is to be increased the product label should be carefully scrutinised to make sure that is does not contain hidden sugar in its formulation.

In the case of diabetes, any product from the health food counter demands the endorsement of the physician providing the diabetic care.

★ *Gold Standard*
• Not established, but fibre may be helpful.

Possibly Useful
• Antioxidant preparations • Vitamin B complex preparations • Gamma linolenic acid preparations.

See also: **Evening Primrose Oil; Fibre; Glossary; Plant Oils; Potassium; Selenium; Vitamins A, B, C and E.**

DYSMENORRHOEA

DYSMENORRHOEA, or painful periods, is one of the commonest symptoms experienced by women. It is also one of the most neglected areas of medical research. Yet not less than 50 per cent of women experience some discomfort as part of menstruation, and 5–10 per cent of all girls in their late teens and early twenties are incapacitated by dysmenorrhoea for at least several hours each month.

Signs and Symptoms

Dysmenorrhoea is commonly experienced for a few hours *before* and *after* the actual period of menstruation, and usually

223

lasts for a total of less than 12 hours each month. The intense spasmodic nature of the pain is characteristic and is felt mainly in the pit of the stomach or in the thighs.

In about 30 per cent of cases dysmenorrhoea does not occur until the periods have been established for two to four years. This usually indicates that the victim has started ovulating (releasing egg cells from the ovaries) regularly, and has become fully fertile. The peak incidence of dysmenorrhoea is between the ages of 18 and 24. French gynaecologists claim that dysmenorrhoea is cured by marriage. Worldwide gynaecological opinion agrees that it is usually cured by childbirth. You don't have to be a genius to put two and two together here!

Orthodox Medical Management

This ranges from the humble hot water bottle to the temporary suppression of ovulation by steroids, similar to those used for oral contraception. Most commonly prescribed, however, are simple painkillers like aspirin and paracetamol and anti-spasmodics, for example Buscopan. All medical treatment is accompanied by variable levels of side effects, and this has led to an exploration of health food-type therapies, but with very little enthusiasm as far as the medical profession is concerned.

Good Health-Food Management

VITAMIN B3 AND DYSMENORRHOEA

A small experimental study was carried out in 1954 when 80 women took niacin in 100mg dosage twice daily for ten days prior to menstruation and then every two to three hours during menstruation. Relief from symptoms occurred in 90 per cent of cases – the effect being enhanced if rutin and ascorbic acid (in 60mg and 300mg doses respectively) were given as well as the niacin. (Rutin is a bioflavonoid, sometimes known as Vitamin P.

VITAMIN E AND DYSMENORRHOEA

Another trial in 1955 was a placebo-controlled study in which 100 victims received either Vitamin E in a 50mg dosage thrice daily or a placebo for ten days premenstrually and for the following 40 days. An advantage of 18 per cent symptom relief was gained for the active treatment over the controls.

MAGNESIUM, PYRIDOXINE AND DYSMENORRHOEA

Magnesium and pyridoxine therapy has proved successful in the management of pre-menstrual tension, and an experimental study has examined similar therapy for dysmenorrhoea. There was a progressive decrease in the intensity and duration of the menstrual cramps, but the relatively high doses of pyridoxine used would not be acceptable today, although no cases of toxicity were reported in the study in question. The combination is perhaps worth trying.

GOOD BUYS

★ *Gold Standard*
• None firmly established but niacin or Vitamin B_3 in 200mg dosage taken daily may be a contender for this position.

Useful
• Vitamin E, 50mg thrice daily.

Worth Trying
• Vitamin B group and magnesium complexes • PRN Mega Multi's (HEALTHCRAFTS) and Confiance (WASSEN).

See also: **Glossary; PMS; Magnesium; Vitamins B, C and E.**

225

ECZEMA AND ALLERGIC DERMATITIS

ECZEMA is Greek for 'to boil out', and to some extent the itchy and weepy rash of eczema, of infants in particular, looks as though something is 'boiling out' of the skin. There are dozens of types of eczema.

Dermatitis means inflammation of the skin. Doctors subdivide dermatitis by a prefix that tells us something about the cause of the dermatitis: solar (sun) dermatitis, chemical dermatitis, sebhorroeic (grease) dermatitis and allergic dermatitis. In this latter case dermatitis tends to blend into eczema.

In many eczemas, allergy is involved. Research carried out in Bristol quite recently revealed that allergy sufferers have as part of their make-up a defect in an important enzyme known as delta-6-desaturase (see Glossary). This is vital for the manufacture of GLA (gamma linolenic acid) in the body, and has led to a new concept of allergy being to some extent a nutritional deficiency disease.

There are several health foods marketed that are rich in this enzyme nutrient, the most popular of which is evening primrose oil.

Sign and Symptoms

Eczema is a rough, red and itchy rash that comes in patches. Often symptoms include heat and redness, swelling, itching or pain and loss of efficient skin function. The skin normally contains the flesh and protects it. If this function is lost, the body fluids tend to ooze out and the skin becomes prone to infection.

As in all allergic states, various trigger factors operate, particularly in infants. Fat babies often get eczema, for instance. In tiny babies it first appears on the forehead and cheeks; in year-olds the nappy area is often affected; in older children the skin crease areas show the itchy rash.

Orthodox Medical Management

Doctors start by organising 'exclusion diets' or prescribing bland, soothing preparations that have few side effects. These are called *emollients* (oily preparations) or *emulsions* (mostly urea preparations). Both tend to bind water to the skin. Creams based on glycerine have a similar function. Lanolin ointments and creams are out of fashion as they can themselves cause allergic reactions. Various anti-itch preparations are used locally on the skin, e.g. camphor or crotamiton ointments. Antihistamines are seldom used locally these days, but are effective as adult anti-itch preparations when taken by mouth. Doctors and pharmacists warn against possible sedative side effects.

If these simple skin remedies are ineffective, preparations containing steroids and/or antibiotics are often prescribed.

Good Health-Food Management

EVENING PRIMROSE OIL AND ECZEMA

Babies and youngsters that suffer from the condition known as infantile eczema often improve rapidly if this vital nutrient is replaced in the diet or rubbed into the skin.

Dosage in all nutritional supplementation often tends to be less precise and less rigid than is common practice when using conventional drugs. The defective intake in young eczema sufferers can usually be made up in older children by 3 × 500mg of evening primrose oil taken daily for several weeks. (Sometimes nausea and indigestion are a side effect.)

Often in the case of babies evening primrose oil rubbed into the skin provides extra sustenance and also acts as a soothing local application. Of late it has become common knowledge that breast-fed babies rarely suffer from infantile eczema and it is possible that the fundamental allergic state is produced because artificial (formula) baby feeds are manufactured from dried cows' milk which is deficient in the vital anti-allergic nutrient.

With adults, the results can be even more remarkable. After

a 12-week hospital trial in which patients took relatively high doses of evening primrose oil (8 – 10 × 500mg capsules daily) there was found to be a dramatic improvement in the takers' skin, and incidentally, a normalisation of the victims' enzyme blood tests when these were repeated.

In another study, 60 adults and 39 children suffering from eczema-dermatitis received either evening primrose oil or placebo (inert similar capsule) for 12 weeks and in various doses ranging between 1 – 3g for adults, and 1 – 2g for children. Itching improved significantly in the evening primrose oil takers at all doses, but higher doses provided greater improvement. This was a double blind, crossover study in which neither patients nor assessing physician knew which patients were receiving test substances and when, and so provides strong evidence of the efficacy of the health food in question.

Doctors are starting to use evening primrose oil products to treat their patients suffering from allergic-type eczema, and EPOgam is now a NHS prescription product in adult and paediatric forms. The manufacturers stress 'use with care in patients suffering from schizophrenia, patients with a history of epilepsy and those taking anti-epilepsy drugs'. These strictures should apply to all products containing gamma-linolenic acid. Rarely, side effects (nausea and headaches) limit use.

GOOD BUYS

★ *Gold Standard*
● Evening primrose oil. For adults, any preparation which can provide 480mg of evening primrose oil (or equivalent), taken twice daily for 8 – 12 weeks.

See also: **Allergy; Glossary; Evening Primrose Oil; Plant Oils.**

FIBROCYSTIC BREAST DISEASE

THIS condition is sometimes referred to as 'the lumpy breast syndrome', and it is characterised by an overgrowth of glandular and fibrous tissue in the breast or breasts. Tenderness that can develop into actual pain is present in some women. Usually multiple lumps occur, but sometimes single cysts occur. Fibrocystic breast disease is a very common disorder, and an idea of how very variable the condition is can best be grasped by an examination of the names under which it has been paraded for years by doctors, health workers and medical journalists. These include fibroadenosis, benign mammary dysplasia, chronic mastitis, cystic mastitis and benign breast disease. Whatever label we pin upon this condition, it is presumed to be caused by fluctuating levels of female sex hormones. It is commonest in women in the 30 to 50 age group.

Signs and Symptoms

Apart from the worrying lumps there is often a feeling of heaviness of the breasts and very occasionally a discharge from the nipple. Symptoms tend to be at their worst during the second half of the menstrual cycle.

In all cases of fibrocystic disease, it is essential for a doctor to rule out breast cancer. If single large cysts develop as part of the disease these are sometimes aspirated (drained of fluid by a syringe and needle) or a biopsy is carried out (removal of a small area of tissue). Sometimes the special radiological diagnostic procedure called mammography is used to differentiate between fibrocystic disease and cancer.

Orthodox Medical Management

Once a firm exclusion of malignancy has been made, medical management may range from reassurance (which is reinforced by regular self-examination of the breast), to a variety of drug

229

treatments including tranquillisers, diuretic drugs (which stimulate an artificial dehydration), painkillers and certain hormone treatments.

Good Health-Food Management

A large observational study that involved 634 women suffering from fibrocystic disease linked it with caffeine intake. The more substantial the intake of caffeine, the greater the incidence of the disease. Coffee contains considerable amounts of caffeine, while tea contains both caffeine and chemically related theophylline; some cola drinks also contain caffeine. When all methylated xanthines (caffeine, theophylline and theobromine – found in cocoa) are excluded from the diet, several studies reported a statistically significant improvement in benign breast disease. When one considers the side effects associated with general medical management of fibrocystic breast disease it would seem logical to try the effect of such a diet. Replacing coffee in the diet with decaffeinated products may go some way towards bringing about this prophylaxis, but several surveys only found convincing improvement in women who totally excluded all of the methylxanthines from their diet.

VITAMINS A AND E IN FIBROCYSTIC BREAST DISEASE

Some studies have reported that Vitamins A and E are beneficial in the treatment of the disease, but patient numbers in trials were small. Regular intake of more than 7500µg of Vitamin A is dangerous for women.

EVENING PRIMROSE OIL AND FIBROCYSTIC BREAST DISEASE

A relatively large experimental study and a double blind study which involved 41 patients found evening primrose oil to be beneficial as far as the pain of fibrocystic disease was concerned. A dosage of 1500µg GLA twice daily was prescribed. (Special care is advised in schizophrenic and epilepsy patients. Nausea and indigestion may be side effects of GLA.)

GOOD BUYS

★ *Gold Standard*
• Evening primrose oil.

Useful
• Vitamin A and E preparations.

See also: **Glossary; PMS; Evening Primrose Oil; Plant Oils; Vitamins A and E.**

GALL BLADDER PROBLEMS

THE gall bladder is part of the digestive system, and acts as the storehouse of bile, a substance which is manufactured by the liver in order to help digest foods. Hard stones, composed of cholesterol, bile pigments and calcium salts, can form in the gall bladder.

Many gallstones are 'silent', and produce no symptoms. When, however, a gallstone tries to escape from the gall bladder by passing down the bile ducts to the intestine, then it can get stuck and irritate and inflame the gall bladder, its ducts or the duct of the nearby pancreas. Cholecystitis or pancreatitis may develop or the patient may also experience an unpleasant attack of gall-bladder colic. Jaundice is also a possible complication.

Gallstones occur most frequently in middle-aged women and older people of both sexes, particularly those who are overweight and have a high level of cholesterol in their blood.

Signs and Symptoms

Severe abdominal, chest or shoulder pain and vomiting may occur. Fever may indicate gall-bladder inflammation a day or two after the initial attack of gall-bladder colic.

Orthodox Medical Management

To some extent this depends on how much of a problem gallstones are to the patient. A single, symptomless stone discovered by chance investigation can often be safely left alone. Once symptoms have occurred then routine medical management includes painkillers, antibiotics, operation or an attempt at dissolving the gallstones with drugs. On a world-wide basis the incidence of gall-bladder disease is enormous. In Britain, gall-bladder surgery remains one of the most common operations performed today.

Good Health-Food Management

Happily, diet and good health foods can play a positive part in the *prevention* of gall bladder disease.

For many years it has been realised that there is a positive relationship between a high intake of refined carbohydrates and gallstones. A *British Medical Journal* report reviewed 267 patients hospitalised for newly-diagnosed gallstones. It compared their sugar intake with that of a similar number of matched controls in the community, and a similar number of other hospital patients. A high sugar intake proved to be a high risk factor independent of obesity, and so the remedy is obvious – eat less sugar.

A diet that is low in fat as well as sugar would seem to be indicated.

FIBRE AND GALLSTONES

In various trials (see page 40), fibre was shown to be both protective against gallstone formulation, and to decrease cholesterol in the bile, presumably because fibre – oat bran in particular – can help protect against over high levels of blood cholesterol.

Reasonable advice is to try an extra 27g fibre per day to escape gallstones.

VITAMIN C AND GALLSTONES

Nutritional research has demonstrated that animals can grow gallstones quite easily if fed on a high-cholesterol diet. But this tendency can be prevented by supplementing the diet with extra Vitamin C.

ESSENTIAL FATTY ACIDS AND GALLSTONES

Something of a surprise finding in animal studies was that the supplementation of the diet with essential fatty acids for a period of between 6 to 12 months is associated with complete or partial dissolution of proven gallstones. The product used was an EFA concentrate marketed as Rowchol. Other EFA concentrates appear on the shelves of health food outlets, and may well prove to be prophylactic as far as gallstones are concerned, but signficant research in this field is awaited. See Glossary.

GOOD BUYS

● High-fibre products that do not contain sugary 'extras' ● Any Vitamin C preparation with a 200mg daily dosage ● Cod liver oil or other EFA concentrates, provided that medical management does not conflict with a low-fat diet.

See also: **Cod Liver Oil; Evening Primrose Oil; Fibre; Glossary; Marine Oils; Plant Oils; Vitamin C.**

GOITRE

GOITRE IS a swelling of the thyroid gland in the neck, which expands as it tries to work harder to manufacture its essential hormone in the face of a dietary deficiency in iodine. Goitre was endemic at the birth of the century in parts of Britain, Europe and the USA, primarily in areas where there was a low soil content of iodine. Today it is a rarity in the West, for it was found that by giving people a little extra mineral iodine in their table salt, goitre could be virtually eliminated, except in certain rare circumstances.

Any goitre must be treated by orthodox medicine, but to ensure there is no lack of iodine in the diet, eat plenty of seafood, perhaps supplementing it with what are known as the sea vegetables – seaweeds such as kelp, carrageen, laver and dulse, and samphire. Kelp tablets are available in healthfood shops.

See also: **Iodine**

HAYFEVER OR ALLERGIC RHINITIS

RHINITIS occurs in three forms: acute (the common cold), chronic or perennial, and allergic – commonly known as hayfever. Hayfever affects some 5–10 per cent of the population. Many victims also suffer from other allergic problems, especially asthma and eczema. The condition runs in families, develops before the age of 30 and affects women more than men. The common allergens or allergic triggers of hayfever, or seasonal rhinitis, are pollens; the allergens of chronic or perennial rhinitis are pollutants (including tobacco smoke), pet hairs and, most important, house dust. Pregnancy and the use of oral contraceptives sometimes trigger hayfever symptoms too, which is very odd.

Signs and Symptoms

These are very familiar as they are similar to those of the common cold – runny nose, runny eyes, sore eyes, catarrh, sore throat, sneezing and coughs.

If they occur in springtime, tree pollens are often implicated; it will be grass pollens after the second week in June; and when autumn symptoms occur they are mostly due to moulds growing invisibly on lawns, compost heaps and on a variety of plants. Some people suffer all year round, due to allergens such as house dust.

Orthodox Medical Management

Conventional treatment using antihistamines is often unsatisfactory, providing temporary relief, but rebound symptoms limit drug use, and habituation may become a problem. Antihistamines can cause drowsiness and are unsafe for those who drive, or who operate machinery. The most effective medical treatments involve the prophylactic cromoglycate, Intal. (Intal is useless therapeutically – it only acts as a preventative, prophylactic measure.) Sometimes steroids are used, but side effects can be worrying. Desensitisation procedures are often disappointing, as is environmental control (avoiding irritants) other than by the regular airing of rooms, beds and duvets.

'Non-medical' treatment involves the elimination of many well-known *food* allergens from the diet. In one group of 197 patients (who had failed hayfever treatment with environmental control), an oligo-allergenic diet (one that induced few allergies) was prescribed. The diet involved eating only rice, olive oil, turkey, lettuce, peeled pears, salt, sugar, water and tea. Some 52 patients improved on this diet, demonstrating that unsuspected food allergy may well be related to hayfever and perennial rhinitis. In other words, if you stop challenging your body with food allergens, it can cope with pollens and dusts.

Good Health-Food Management

Vitamin C and zinc supplements have been used in cases of hayfever, but it would seem that, generally speaking, hayfever is not otherwise much helped by health foods. The products offered for hayfever in health food outlets – Antifect (Potters), Cantassium Hayfever Remedy, Bioforce Pollinoson, Nelson's Hayfever Tablets – are unproven remedies and cannot be medically endorsed with any enthusiasm.

Worth Considering
• Over-the-counter antihistamine remedies.

See also: **Allergy; Colds; Eczema; Herbalist Products; Homoeopathic Products.**

HERPES

EXPERTS on viruses tell us that the herpes virus is one of the oldest viruses known to attack humankind: it has apparently been doing so for around a million years.

Herpes means 'to creep' and a characteristic of the herpes virus is to produce blisters that spread slowly on your skin (creep), burst and produce a highly infectious fluid that fulfils the virus's main ambition – to infect another person. The virus exists in three principal forms, as *Herpes simplex* types 1 and 2, and *Herpes zoster*.

The *Herpes simplex* virus (type 1) has infected most of us by the time we reach adulthood as an unremembered minor childhood ailment; in this type cold sores tend to appear around the mouth from time to time as a 'reminder' of that childhood ailment. *Herpes simplex* virus (type 2) is the usual cause of a sexually transmitted disease; it too is characterized by blisters, but on the genitals. Both types of *Herpes simplex* infections tend to recur from time to time, particularly when the immune system is compromised or under stress. In other words you can get herpes if you have a cold, or if you develop pneumonia, or simply if you are run down. Some women get cold sores when their period comes; exposure to sunlight or cold can activate them as well.

Herpes zoster is what is commonly known as shingles, and it is most usually seen in older people who have had chickenpox in childhood (the virus has lain dormant in the nervous system). A rash appears on the chest, accompanied by fever, and quite often by considerable pain in the nerves along which the rash lies.

Orthodox Medical Management

This is variable and depends on the type of infection, the site of infection and its severity. It can range from a dab of calamine lotion to the most exotic antiviral medicines, for example the antiviral drug Acylovir.

Good Health-Food Management

Because conventional medical management is frequently disappointing, remedies from the health-food counter have gained in popularity.

VITAMIN C AND *HERPES SIMPLEX*

A mixture of Vitamin C and bioflavonoids was evaluated on an experimental double blind basis (200mg of each were given thrice daily) on the first signs of a herpes relapse in a group of recurrent herpes sufferers. Compared with a placebo, the duration of the herpes attack decreased from nine days to exactly half that time.

ZINC AND *HERPES SIMPLEX*

Zinc has been shown in experimental studies to inhibit herpes virus replication. (The herpes virus reproduces in a curious way. Once inside a living cell it takes charge of the cell's internal biochemistry and switches all the cell's bio-energy from its normal function and commands it instead to produce virus particles which can then infect other healthy cells. This process is called replication.) Trials in Australia and elsewhere have been most impressive, both of zinc taken internally and applied locally (see Zinc).

PROPOLIS AND *HERPES ZOSTER*

Propolis, the substance that bees use as a sealant in their hives, has been applied as a tincture, with some success, to relieve the pain of shingles (see Pollen, Propolis and Royal Jelly).

AMINO ACIDS (LYSINE) AND HERPES

Lysine is believed to help prevent and reduce the duration of an attack of cold sores. An experimental crossover study was encouraging, but double blind trials are negative.

GOOD BUYS

● Zinc sulphate ointment and zinc tablets ● Vitamin C with bioflavonoids (QUEST)

Worth Trying
● Laboprin (LAB), lysine and aspirin sachets.

See also: **Glossary; Pollen, Propolis and Royal Jelly; Vitamin C; Zinc.**

HYPERKINESIS (HYPERACTIVITY)

DR Spock, the father of paediatrics, did not even mention hyperkinesis, or hyperactivity in children, whereas nowadays it is taken quite seriously. It has even been re-named recently, as Attention Deficit Disorder (ADD).

Although for several years there has been a sneaking suspicion that hyperkinesis was a food-linked disease, the possibility that diet modification and health-food supplementation was a feasible and worthy method of managing this upsetting family problem is only slowly being realized.

Some 5–15 per cent of children suffer to some extent, six times as many boys as girls. The fact that girls are so much less affected is puzzling, but one expert on micronutrients, Professor Derek Bryce-Smith, believes that this is because the brain biochemistry in women is fundamentally different from that of men.

Signs and Symptoms

One expert has defined hyperkinesis recently as a condition characterised by a child's inability to keep still. The victim is constantly fidgeting, has poor concentration, a short attention span and rapid mood changes. Unpredictable, often aggressive behaviour and a surly expression on the part of the child is common. Excessive frustration also characterises the condition. Many hyperkinetic children have sleep problems, too. They often seem to experience a raging thirst at times. Such children often seem permanently unhappy and unhealthy, or chronically depressed. At school, teachers complain that they never finish any allotted task properly, and there is often an associated dyslexia (word blindness).

The fundamental cause of ADD is thought by some to be lack of oxygen, infection or trauma at or around the time of birth. To identify whether a child may have ADD, or is simply naughty, see the box on page 240.

ADD OR SIMPLY NAUGHTY?

Inattention

At least three of the following suggest ADD:

1. Often fails to finish things started
2. Often does not listen to instructions
3. Easily distracted
4. Difficulty in concentrating
5. Difficulty in sticking to a play activity

Impulsivity

At least three of the following suggest ADD:

1. Acts before thinking
2. Shifts excessively from one activity to the next
3. Difficulty in organising any work task
4. Needs a lot of supervision
5. Frequently calls out in class
6. Difficulty in taking turns

Hyperactivity

At least two of the following suggest ADD:

1. Runs about or climbs excessively
2. Difficulty in sitting still, or excessive fidgeting
3. Difficulty in staying seated
4. Restless sleeper
5. Appears driven – is always on the go.

Is Food the Trigger?

Many believe that a food deficiency or a food allergy may be responsible for hyperkinesis, but to some extent the question remains unanswered. Slowly, however, paediatricians seem to be moving towards a consensus. One consultant paediatrician studied a group of 400 children with behavioural and learning difficulties, and found that certain dietary *exclusions* were the only therapeutic manoeuvres that paid real dividends. Junk foods, which are rich in chemical additives, were excluded from the diet, together with common food allergens (including cola drinks, coffee, chocolate, artificial sweeteners, bacon, ham and Continental-type sausages), all take-away foods, and highly sugary and fatty foods.

Foods that have been proved to be unlikely to provoke an allergic response – for example, lamb, pears, turkey, wholemeal bread, fish, cheese (if not cows' milk), potatoes, rice, beans, green and root vegetables, lentils and fresh fruit – formed the basis of revised everyday eating.

High sugar intake has been suspected as a cause of hyperkinesis. But in studies that looked at groups of hospitalised, behaviourally disturbed children, in which high-sucrose diets have been compared with low-sucrose diets, no significant differences between the level of disturbed behaviour could be observed between the groups. So it would therefore seem unlikely that sweets as such are very much involved in producing hyperkinesis.

When, however, over-active children are treated with oligo-antigenic diets in well-designed, double blinded, crossover trials (oligo-antigenic diets are very low in foods implicated in any type of food allergy), children improved. When allergy-linked foods were reintroduced, their symptoms returned or worsened. (That there may be links between diet and delinquent behaviour generally has recently been considered seriously enough for the UK charity, Natural Justice, to be awarded a £20,000 Government grant to research a connection between diet and anti-social behaviour in the UK.)

Orthodox Medical Management

In severe cases a psychotherapeutic approach is necessary. Generally speaking, conventional medicine has little to offer in most cases other than dietary measures.

Good Health-Food Management

When one considers the great difficulties that confront a family with a hyperkinetic child, and the general lack of success that many prescription remedies, psychiatric treatment and hospitalisation bring in such cases, it is perhaps quite amazing that greater emphasis on dietary rearrangement and supplementation with health foods is not given greater credence in hyperkinesis.

VITAMINS AND HYPERKINESIS

In one experimental single blind study (where the assessors are aware of the nature of the medication, but not the participants), 100 hyperkinetic children were given mega doses of various B complex vitamins or a placebo as part of their everyday diet. About 15 per cent of the children responded favourably to pyridoxine (B_6), 8 per cent to thiamin (B_1) and several to nicotinamide (niacin, or B_3). In another study 33 children with disturbed behaviour were treated with nicotinamide and Vitamin C in mega doses. Only one child failed to respond to the therapy, and all relapsed when a placebo was substituted for the vitamins.

EVENING PRIMROSE OIL AND HYPERKINESIS

Hyperkinesis has been linked with foods which inhibit prostaglandin conversion in the body, which suggests a lack of essential fatty acids (see Glossary). Some studies have been mounted and good results are being reported after supplementation with evening primrose oil.

GOOD BUYS

• Vitamin B complex (SEVEN SEAS) • Compleat Vitamin B (HEALTHCRAFTS) • Vitamin C • Evening primrose oil supplements.

See also: **Evening Primrose Oil; Glossary; Plant Oils; Vitamins B and C.**

HYPERTENSION

HYPERTENSION, or high blood pressure, is a curious condition in many ways. First of all, blood pressure is a continuous variable in all of us, and in the large majority of cases no cause can be found for *high* blood pressure. (In rather less than 10 per cent of cases of hypertension a cause can be identified, and in these, abnormalities in the kidneys are fundamentally responsible.) It is often difficult to define when someone's blood pressure is 'high' because the level at which high blood pressure causes *symptoms* or disease varies so much with age, sex, race and country.

For life insurance purposes a blood pressure with a diastolic level of 105mm Hg or above is considered to be a hypertensive level in the UK. Blood pressure is normally expressed as a double figure, say 150/90, the higher figure reflecting the blood pressure when the heart is contracting (systole), while the lower figure is the continuous background level of blood pressure when the heart's ventricles are relaxed (diastole). The World Health Organisation takes 160/95 as a level of normalcy. In the large US (Framingham) studies, 160/95 is deemed abnormal and 140/90 to 165/95 is regarded as borderline.

Your size and shape come into it, and obesity is associated with hypertension. What you eat is important, too. A low salt intake protects you to some extent against hypertension. A low fat intake protects both against obesity, and also against cholesterol being deposited in the arteries: if these narrow, the heart has to work harder to pump blood through them.

Hypertension is extremely common, affecting 10–20 per cent of the adult population in the UK. Your doctor is the best person to diagnose whether or not you are hypertensive.

Signs and Symptoms

Usually there are none! Nosebleeds and headaches – long thought to be symptoms of hypertension – are no more or less frequent in the hypertensive. Untreated severe hypertension can produce secondary symptoms – e.g. angina, breathlessness, heart failure and stroke illness – once the persistent hypertension damages the arteries.

Orthodox Medical Management

General 'fitness' measures, including reduction of obesity, reduction of heavy alcohol intake, salt restriction and sensible exercise and relaxation regimes are part and parcel of more detailed medical management of hypertension.

Drug treatments of hypertension are effective but have usually to be faced on a long-term basis, and side effects of the drugs commonly used in hypertensive therapy are often a problem. Often the drug selected has to be modified in an attempt to evade unacceptable side effects. Three main classes of drugs are currently used: diuretics, beta-blockers and vasodilators (see Glossary).

Medical treatment of hypertension is enthusiastically prescribed by doctors because hypertension is associated with an increased risk of stroke illness, coronary artery disease and heart failure.

Good Health-Food Management

Vegetarian diets have been widely demonstrated to be profoundly beneficial in lowering blood pressure in many well-designed controlled trials reported in the most prestigious of the world's medical journals. But it is difficult to decide *exactly what* in the diet is bringing about the much-desired effect, for vegetable diets are also high in fibre, in polyunsaturate content, and in potassium and magnesium intake.

The Finns have most unenviable death rates from hypertension and heart disease. Several well-documented studies have demonstrated that when Finns change their eating habits and eat less saturated fat and more polyunsaturated fat, they reduce their blood pressure quite significantly.

MARINE OILS AND HYPERTENSION

The possibility of other health foods being useful in the management of hypertension seems to have revolved around a search for 'missing' nutrients in the average diet of us human omnivores. One double blind crossover study examined the effects of a marine oil (MAXEPA) on hypertension, and it was found to reduce blood pressure by about 5 per cent compared to a placebo. But the reduction in diastolic BP (thought by most doctors to be the most important measurement) was not of statistical significance.

MINERALS AND HYPERTENSION

Magnesium, in many ways a mysterious substance as far as our health is concerned, has been investigated in the management of hypertension with largely negative results. But potassium supplementation has been shown, in an experimental double blind crossover study, to significantly lower the blood pressure, by restoring the correct sodium/potassium balance. However, market forces discourage pharmaceutical companies from mounting large magnesium or potassium trials. Potassium supplementation was once, of course, part and parcel of orthodox medical management of certain types of diuretic therapy. These drugs produced an excessive loss of potassium from the body, but now potassium-sparing diuretics have been introduced.

FIBRE AND HYPERTENSION

Health-food shoppers rarely get involved specifically in scientific research, but an exception to this rule occurred recently when 300 health food shop customers each agreed to supplement their diet with an extra 100g (4oz) of fibre per week. After a trial period their blood pressure was found to have fallen by 4 and 3mm Hg (systolic and diastolic). This small reduction is definitely worthwhile if it displaces someone from a high or borderline group, especially when it seems likely that for men aged 40 or over each rise of 10mm Hg increases the risk of heart disease by 20 per cent.

GARLIC AND HYPERTENSION

Perhaps the most modern and certainly most promising newcomer to the small group of health-food troops that we can muster in the fight against hypertension is associated more often with the greengrocer's than the health-food shop or pharmacy – garlic. Many trials have demonstrated its undoubted efficacy (see Garlic).

HYPERTENSION MANAGEMENT

Health-food management of hypertension would seem to centre around the following six-point plan:

1. Increase fibre intake to the extent of an extra 100g (4oz) fibre per week. **Good Buys:** Jordan's Oat Bran, Shredded Wheat, All-Bran, other bran products.

2. Take a marine oil supplement daily. Modest therapeutic claims support this.

3. Make modest increases in potassium intake, preferably in the form of extra fruit and vegetables.

4. Reduce salt intake but beware of *high*-potassium salt substitutes which may ease the unfit into potassium intoxication. Herbal salt substitutes rather than high-potassium products are to be preferred. **Good Buy:** St Giles Foods Herbal Salt Replacer.

5. Eat garlic regularly or take garlic products.

6. Reduce high-calorie foods, especially fat.

See also: **Artery Problems; Cardiac Problems; Tension and Stress; Cod Liver Oil; Fibre; Garlic; Magnesium; Marine Oils; Potassium.**

IMMUNODEPRESSION

THE most devastating demonstration of immunodepression is the state of total health failure that eventually occurs in AIDS – the acquired immunodeficiency syndrome – in which all of the complex systems that fuel the normal immune response collapse, with tragic results. There are, however, less serious failures of the immune response or system – when you just feel 'run down' or maybe catch cold after cold.

AIDS is, of course, a specific disease wrought on the body's complex immune system by a virus. But it is known that malnutrition of various types can also depress the immune system. Tuberculosis, for instance, was rife in Europe during the later years of the Second World War, and declined rapidly in many countries, including Britain, as the nations escaped from their war-footing nutritional economies. This was well in advance of the introduction of modern, potent anti-tuberculosis drugs.

Over 50 years ago the Ministry of Food in Britain took its nutritional policies very seriously – a fact that was referred to recently in *The Times* (10.4.91), when Britain's leading gastroenterologist, Sir Francis Avery Jones, called for a revival of governmental endorsement of 'protective foods'. Sir Francis drew attention to the often-ignored micronutrients, which he rightly sees as 'lubricants for the thousands of enzyme chemical reactions which affect every cell of the body and sustain life. It is their availability which makes all the difference between feeling below par and on top of the world, ensuring vitality and extra energy. They determine the strength of our defence against infections, almost certainly inhibit the damage by excess fat to the coronary arteries in the heart, and are thought to arrest early pre-cancer changes.'

Gradually a change has been taking place in the attitude that doctors and scientists are taking towards the nutritional needs of the individual. Two sorts of nutritional scientist have recently been identified. First of all, there is the classical nutritionalist who only believes in a crude sort of absolute evidence of nutritional need. For instance, if you give people no Vitamin C they will eventually develop scurvy, or if you give them no iodine in their diet, they will develop the nasty neck swellings we call goitres. In our Western world today there are few examples of these *absolute* deficiency states occurring, although 'borderline' deficiencies – scurvy and another nutritional disease, rickets – keep cropping up in the world's medical journals.

The second type of nutritional scientist does not think it right and proper to cling too tightly to this 'flat-earth' policy related to nutrition – mainly because such a policy means that large numbers of people are flirting with diseases like coronary heart disease and certain cancers. These 'round-earth' nutritionists are reacting positively and advocating supplementation with health foods of various types as indicated in this good health food guide.

Signs and Symptoms

The signs and symptoms of AIDS are extremely varied and include acute and chronic infections, generalised glandular enlargement, lassitude, fever, weight loss, dementia, various malignancies and chronic diarrhoea.

However, few readers of this section will be looking for a cure for AIDS or a defence against the handful of specific immunodeficiency diseases that are only rather slowly being recognised by doctors. But there are many of us who feel too often that we are in less than perfect health. Maybe you feel you have too many colds. Perhaps you are prone to mild, but debilitating infections, or tire over-easily. There is a condition that has obtained a fair amount of medical publicity called the *post-viral syndrome*, in which, after a 'flu-like illness, or perhaps an attack of one of the common infectious diseases, the sufferer is left in a chronic state of what is best described as debility. They tire easily and find it difficult to get down to anything. Sometimes this leads to long-term unemployment as the victims seem to abdicate from everyday life, so generally but vaguely ill do they feel. A medical check-up is always necessary in such conditions, but people who suffer from any chronic 'nameless' condition soon, it seems, lose the kind concern and helpful attention that doctors give to 'genuinely' sick people.

Orthodox Medical and Good Health-Food Management

It is becoming possible to measure and appraise the immune response, an intricate and somewhat esoteric subspeciality in modern medicine, and so for the first time to explore the possibility of developing substances that can alter the immune response in a positive way. (To a large extent knowledge has developed fastest with methods of *suppressing* the immune response – a process vitally necessary to combat tissue rejection in organ transplant surgery.)

All the cells involved in the immune response are derived from the bone marrow. The lymphocytes are the largest single group of these cells and occur in various forms. The so-called T-lymphocytes are involved in cell-mediated immunity while the B-lymphocytes are involved in non-cellular immunity responses. Neutrophil cells are the largest group of white cells – they have a very short life span (of 6–20 hours) and play a primary role in non-specific immunity by engulfing and digesting germs.

It is worthwhile just making a fleeting acquaintance with these intricacies because most of the interesting work being carried out on nutrients and immunity involves investigating how you react as far as this complex nest of specialized cells is concerned. For instance, after a week's dosage of beta-carotene (in an 80mg daily dosage) there is an increased number of T-lymphocytes circulating in your blood, indicating an enhanced immune response. Deficiency of Vitamin A in your body has been shown to reduce the response to an antigen challenge, demonstrating reduced immunity. A large dose (500mg daily) of Vitamin C has been demonstrated to enhance the response of T-lymphocytes in the elderly, in a controlled trial situation. In other words, it enhances their immunity. Simple iron deficiency (relatively common in children and the elderly) has been shown to impair the immune response, especially when associated with lack of selenium and Vitamin E in the diet.

The main nutritional substances that immunology has identified as being beneficial, however, are the antioxidant Vitamins A (beta-carotene), C and E, together with the micronutrient selenium. So great has been the recent interest in the antioxidant substances that a large international conference met in London in 1989 to explore the subject at great length and also in considerable depth. This heralded a new era of interest in protective nutrients.

It seems only sensible, therefore, for those who suffer from any form of immunodepression, or from conditions in which they feel run down and wretched, to try the effects of dietary supplements that contain all the antioxidant nutrients in meaningful doses taken over a reasonably long timescale. If the symptoms are due to long-term malabsorption of nutrients, it may well be a relatively long-term process to adjust the nutritional *status quo* back into rude health once again. Such supplements are readily available and at a reasonable price from reputable manufacturers.

GOOD BUYS

- Multi-antioxidant products, e.g. Selenium-ACE (WASSEN)
- Beta-carotene products ● Vitamin C and E products.

See also: **Colds; Glossary; Tiredness and Fatigue and Iron; Selenium; Vitamins A, C and E.**

INSOMNIA

COMPLAINTS about various types of poor sleep are among the most common heard in the doctor's surgery. Women suffer more than men in this way; the elderly more than the young; and thin people more than fat. Anxiety arising out of the problems of everyday life is often a cause of insomnia.

Although most doctors will say that insomnia does not matter, and that we all get the amount of sleep we need, research does not entirely confirm this. A project that logged the sleep habits of over 1 million North Americans found that those who slept markedly more or less than an average 7 – 8 hours subsequently experienced a raised mortality rate. Depressive illness is associated often with one particular type of insomnia – early-morning waking.

Signs and Symptoms

It is important to differentiate between various types of insomnia, for this can dictate sensible management. There are 'can't get to sleep' types, or 'wake early' types, and insomnia due to pain or anxiety.

Orthodox Medical Management

Drugs are used extensively to treat insomnia. Modern sleeping pills of the diazepam type are safer than the previously popular barbiturates, but side effects are a problem, and habituation occurs if they are abused. A good general principle to ensure a good night's sleep is to precede bedtime with a quiet and regular routine, feeling satisfied that you have done your best with your day, accepting your failures and disabilities while being forgiving of others!

Good Health-Food Management

There is evidence that a pre-bedtime non-stimulating drink, be it malted milk or a herbal tea, promotes sleep – maybe because it reinforces the pre-sleep bedtime routine.

Calcium is also highly thought of as a help for insomnia. Milk contains a great deal of calcium, which is known to induce muscle relaxation, so may well help induce relaxed sleep. Several herbalist products contain herbs which have been considered over the years as calmants or tranquillisers.

One specific health food – L-Tryptophan taken in a 1g dose 30–45 minutes before bedtime, with sugar (but avoiding protein food) – had a health-food reputation that was based on controlled studies and was reported at an American Medical Association Symposium in 1985. It produces a 50 per cent reduction in sleep latency (time to go to sleep), does not interfere with sleep stages, and there were negligible side effects. 'Severe' insomniacs needed larger doses (up to 15g). L-Tryptophan has been used to treat insomniac babies in suitably small doses. Unfortunately, Tryptophan is no longer available as one manufacturer's product was found to have totally unacceptable side effects, and the drug was withdrawn. UK- and US-manufactured Tryptophan was never implicated, however.

GOOD BUYS

- Horlicks and malted bedtime drinks.

Worth considering
- Herbalist products and remedies   • Calcium products.

See also: **Tension and Stress; Calcium; Herbalist Products.**

IRRITABLE BOWEL SYNDROME

SOMETIMES gastroenterologists link this condition with another diagnosis – of non-ulcer dyspepsia – for there is a degree of dyspepsia (wind, nausea, heartburn, upset stomach and vague and changeable patterns of abdominal pain) in which no ulceration in the stomach or duodenum can be discovered on investigation. Some doctors now consider the irritable bowel syndrome (IBS) to be a disease in its own right. This is a reasonable enough attitude, for well over half of all the patients who attend gastroenterology clinics for investigation finish up with the diagnosis of IBS!

Signs and Symptoms

IBS sufferers will probably complain of most of the following symptoms. Usually pain is experienced in the lower left-hand side of the abdomen, but not always. Usually this pain is relieved by the passing of wind or by the opening of the bowels. Often there is a feeling that there is an incomplete emptying of the rectum when the bowels have moved. True watery diarrhoea is unusual. Often the symptoms are chronic and relapsing, but there are usually long symptom-free intervals. Often victims remember episodes of abdominal pain in childhood, and were perhaps diagnosed as suffering from 'abdominal migraine' as children. Despite their complaints, IBS patients look well but may appear rather sad and depressed. Usually they are in under-50 age groups. Good doctors take IBS symptoms seriously and investigate them with kindly interest to exclude other diagnoses that overlap with the symptomatology of IBS.

Orthodox Medical Management

Most gastroenterologists consider that the exclusion of cancer, diverticulitis, ulcers, gall-bladder disease and hiatus hernia, together with the unmasking of depressive illness, to be their prime function in IBS management. Sometimes an antispasmodic drug such as Mebeverine is prescribed, as are some tranquillisers.

Good Heath-Food Management

The cornerstone of medical management is the prescription of fibre in various forms, and here once again orthodox medicine and health foods meet. However, because IBS symptoms come and go, the results of some studies are less than entirely satisfactory.

One therapeutic avenue explored with reference to IBS was to seek out and eliminate or treat food allergy as a possible cause. Once again, results have been equivocal.

Perhaps the most encouraging therapy for IBS involves the taking of a health food in the form of enteric-coated capsules of peppermint oil. Peppermint oil is a relaxer of the smooth muscle complexes that are concerned with the passage of nutrients through the bowel. One double blind study reported in the *British Medical Journal* found peppermint oil capsules to be effective in IBS management. Bowel habit is unchanged on peppermint oil therapy, and it would seem likely that peppermint oil products will feature permanently in IBS management in the future.

GOOD BUYS

★ *Gold Standard*
● Mintec (NOVEX) ● Colpermin sustained-release peppermint oil capsules (Tillots Laboratories).

Worth Trying
● Herbalist peppermint products, and herbal mint teas ● If food allergy is suspected, gluten-free cereal products such as Foodwatch International gluten-free Muesli and Allergy-Aware Rice Bran ● Bran products.

See also: **Fibre; Herbalist Products.**

KIDNEY STONES

KIDNEY stone is a common and potentially serious disease, which can strike one down at any time, but a considerable degree of prevention does seem to be possible these days. The vast majority of kidney stones contain calcium, mostly in the form of phosphates or oxalates, and sometimes even a mixture of the two. Rarer types of stone are made of uric acid or cystine.

The food we eat contains all the elements of kidney stones, and so, in a way, they all come from food. The calcium in them comes mostly from milk and dairy produce, the oxalates from rhubarb, fruits and vegetables, especially spinach and asparagus. Phosphates are present in most of the foods we eat, and so is uric acid and cystine. So why don't we all suffer?

In the search for something in the nature of a trigger factor for kidney stones, all sorts of interesting things have been suggested. There are a couple of tiny glands which sit on top of our thyroid glands (called the parathyroid glands) and sometimes these become overactive. One of the problems which this hyper-parathyroidism produces is kidney stones. But only very rarely is there parathyroid disease in stone victims. Certain bone diseases, such as rickets, osteitis and osteomalacia, are also associated with kidney stones. But again, most stone sufferers are free of these diseases. Finally, kidney infection or anything that interferes with the normal outflow of urine predisposes eventually towards stone formation, but very few stone sufferers are faced with such problems either.

In the majority of cases of kidney stone, none of the pre-disposing causes of stone formation seem relevant, and the stones just come. And when they do come they signal their arrival in various unpleasant ways.

Signs and Symptoms

Sometimes the stone may be passed out from the kidney into the ureter (which connects the kidney to the bladder); this brings on a nasty attack of pain that starts in the loin or the small of the back and then radiates down into the groin. With luck, the stone finds its way into the bladder and may then stay there or may be voided or passed in the urine.

Some kidney stones announce their presence in other ways. For instance, they cause local damage to the urinary tract and blood appears in the urine. If they obstruct the flow of urine, urinary infection may follow, and a sufferer is liable to run a temperature due to an infected urinary tract and have pain.

Orthodox Medical Management

Doctors are always most anxious to preserve kidney health, for kidney damage can be a very serious business indeed, and so they enthusiastically investigate the potential stone victims using various X-rays and other investigative laboratory tests. Sometimes kidney stones need to be removed – which means surgery in most cases – but there is a new method of treatment that persuades kidney and bladder stones to 'explode' into small passable pieces due to ultrasonic shock-wave treatments.

Cutting for stone – the surgical removal of stones – was one of the earliest surgical operations to become fashionable in past centuries, but it is becoming less commonplace today.

Diet and Kidney Stone Formation

In the 1950s it was realised that our kidneys contain microscopic deposits of calcium in them, which it is thought the body removes naturally. When the kidney forms stones it is thought that these mini-stones, or *microliths* as they are called, suddenly decide for some reason to grow. In humans, low-magnesium diets result in a low level of magnesium in the urine, and this tends to make oxalates in the urine become relatively insoluble. Calcium oxalate stones start to form quite easily on an experimental diet low in calcium, low in magnesium and low in Vitamins A and D.

Over 25 years ago an editorial in the *British Medical Journal* drew its readers' attention to the fact that kidney stones were on the increase in Finland, Central Europe, Sweden and Japan, and pointed out that those areas of high calcium/oxalate kidney stone incidence coincided with areas in which there was also a rising incidence of cardiovascular disease.

In 1975, it was pointed out dramatically, in a map of the USA, that in the areas where the water was softest the incidence of kidney stones in the population was highest. Medical geographers were soon to trace a 'kidney-stone belt' across the USA. It included South Carolina and the south-eastern states, which are all soft-water areas, while the Mid-West and South-West earned themselves the epithet of being 'good kidney country'. As more US physicians delved into this somewhat astonishing relationship, the more definitely it became defined. Nebraska, a Mid-Western state well-known for the cardiac health of its inhabitants (it enjoys the lowest incidence of sudden death from coronary disease in the USA), also had the lowest frequency of urinary stones; its water was hard. Finally, a US expert on the subject of kidney stones went on record in 1976 as saying that a statistically significant relationship between kidney stones and the relative softness or hardness of the drinking water had been finally demonstrated.

Some medical geographers have drawn further conclusions relevant to this whole problem that explain seemingly strange and complex variations in kidney-stone incidence on a time-scale basis. Shortly after the First World War, a high incidence of kidney stone occurred in Europe. This coincided with the first use of artificial fertilisers: in farming areas that were low in soil magnesium to start with, the fertilisers caused fields yielding low-magnesium crops to yield even lower-magnesium crops.

Good Health-Food Management

There are a couple of health foods which can benefit kidney-stone sufferers.

MAGNESIUM AND KIDNEY STONES

Doctors working at the US's famous Johns Hopkins Hospital have shown that if magnesium is added to the urine of kidney-stone victims, and subsequently cultured with live connective tissue (a procedure thought to mimic natural stone formation in the body), it loses its ability to produce crystals. Experiments on patients, rather than in test tubes, followed. Supplementary magnesium was given to a group of patients who repeatedly passed urine containing crystals of calcium oxalate – people at high risk of developing kidney stones. On this treatment their condition rapidly improved. Giving extra magnesium to actual urinary stone victims was shown to inhibit both high urinary calcium excretion and new stone formation.

VITAMIN B$_6$ AND KIDNEY STONES

There is some evidence that Vitamin B$_6$ inhibits kidney stone formation, too. The *Journal of the American Medical Association*, in 1965, reported research on a combination of Vitamin B$_6$ and magnesium supplement given to a series of 50 patients suffering from recurrent kidney stone problems. It brought about a reduction of stone relapses. Subsequent surveys have produced similar results.

GOOD BUYS

- Magnesium OK (WASSEN) • Synergistic Magnesium (QUEST)
- Vitamin B$_6$ products.

See also: **Cardiac Problems; Magnesium; Vitamin B$_6$.**

MENOPAUSAL PROBLEMS

HOW women look upon the menopause depends to a large extent upon their previous experience of reproductive life. If painful, heavy periods or premenstrual tension have been a problem of magnitude, the menopause appears as a golden horizon. If too-bountiful fertility has been a worry, the climacteric, or change, is anticipated with pleasure, too.

Basically menopause is the final step in an inevitable and natural part of female life – the gradual loss of the ability to bear children. The climacteric – this whole process of diminishing fertility – begins some ten years before the menopause, and can continue for up to ten years afterwards. This is when the balance of the hormones circulating in the woman's body changes and female hormones finally cease to be secreted by the ovaries.

If there was nothing more to the menopause than the end of menstruation, probably few women would worry about it. But other changes occur at this time, which, together with the cessation of the menses, are often cause for anxiety. However, there is a certain amount of evidence pointing to the fact that many of the more pronounced symptoms are avoidable if the menopause is approached without undue fear and trepidation. For the statistics show that only about one woman in ten is severely affected by the menopause.

Signs and Symptoms

The 'change of life' varies greatly. For the majority of women there is a gradual diminution of the monthly periods. Quite often a period is missed, then the regular cycle is restored for a few months; in time another period or two is missed. This scheme of things repeats itself until finally menstruation stops for good. Among a minority of women, the periods cease abruptly and simply never return. For some women heavy periods usher in the menopause (see also Menorrhagia).

Most important in relation to the menopause is that any

bleeding *afterwards* should be the signal for immediate medical consultation, for post-menopausal bleeding is definitely abnormal.

The age at which the menopause occurs is also widely variable. During the middle of the last century it occured at about 45, and nowadays the average lies between the ages of 45 and 50.

The severity of symptoms probably depends on how abruptly the various hormone changes occur. It used to be assumed that after the menopause the non-functioning of the ovaries was responsible for the symptoms. But now medical opinion admits that it does not understand the mechanisms of production of many of the features of the climacteric.

The most common symptom is, of course, hot flushes. These may simply be a hotness of the face or neck, perhaps spreading over the body. Like blushes, they are frequently triggered by emotional stimuli. Sometimes they are associated with a feeling of choking, palpitations and a sense of being hot and bothered. They usually last a few minutes and may occur in a wide range of frequency – from once a day to once every half hour. In some more severe cases, they occur at night, waking the sufferer up, who may be perspiring excessively and have to change sheets and night clothes.

Orthodox Medical Management

Hormone replacement therapy has made an enormous contribution to the diminishment of menopausal symptoms. Two female sex hormones, an oestrogen and a progesterone, are usually given as a medical treatment known commonly as HRT. This is usually prescribed initially for two to five years; and repeated regular tests are conducted. These include weight and blood-pressure checks, breast and pelvic examinations, cervical smears and sometimes a biopsy test (in which a small particle of the lining of the womb is removed for microscopic examination).

HRT is enthusiastically acclaimed by some women while others reject it, because a light menstrual period from time to time is usually part and parcel of the altered hormonal status.

Understandably, too, some women don't like the idea of taking (artificial) hormones for years on end. There is also a fairly large group of women for whom HRT is not advisable on medical grounds, and this includes heavy smokers, thrombosis and stroke victims, the severely hypertensive, those with liver disease, and women who have had cancer of the breast or uterus.

Good Health-Food Management

Until recently women who were disinclined to take HRT were obliged to 'sit out' a miserable menopause, and had little to comfort them. Nutritional therapy is, however, a relatively simple alternative, is safe, and worthy of a trial.

VITAMIN E AND MENOPAUSAL PROBLEMS

At least four experimental trials, involving over 170 women, have been conducted in which Vitamin E has been shown to be helpful in the management of the menopause. In these trials, doses of between 10 and 100mg were given to menopausal women. (Very few adverse reactions to Vitamin E are recorded.) In the largest trial, which involved 66 women suffering from the vasomotor (hot flush) variety of symptoms, and which was carried out on a single blind study design, very nearly half of the participants had good to excellent results, and a further 16 had fair results. A prompt recurrence of symptoms occurred when a placebo was substituted for the Vitamin E.

It is curious, perhaps, that these trials have been allowed to pass unnoticed by the medical profession. (Of course, legal restrictions prevent health food manufacturers making any claim for Vitamin E in the management of the menopause, as they do for any illnesses.)

CALCIUM AND MENOPAUSAL PROBLEMS

The hormonal upheaval at this time can lead to a diminishment of bone metabolism, leading often to the bone disease of osteoporosis in post-menopausal women. Calcium supplementation could be advisable. There is evidence that HRT minimises menopausal osteoporosis.

GINSENG AND MENOPAUSAL PROBLEMS

Ginseng has earned itself quite a considerable reputation in the health-food management of menopausal problems. This is probably due to its 'adaptogen' properties – enhancing the sufferer's coping skills – but may also be related to the many hormone-like constituents of ginseng.

GOOD BUYS

- A Vitamin E, mineral and antixodant complex.
- Confiance (WASSEN)

Worth Trying
- Menopace (VITABIOTICS) • Ginseng products • Calcium products.

See also: **Dysmenorrhoea; Menorrhagia; PMS; Calcium; Ginseng; Vitamin E.**

MENORRHAGIA

THIS is the medical term for heavy periods. It is applied to a menstrual cycle that is regular enough, but during which more blood is lost than is usual, or perhaps one in which the bleeding continues for longer than is usual.

Menorrhagia is a symptom not a disease. The excessive loss of blood can be due to the internal surface of the womb being over-large (due to fibroids); a local congestion can be the cause; rarely, a blood disorder is involved. Another sort of abnormal blood loss is too-frequent periods – this is usually due to ovary malfunction.

Signs and Symptoms

The reasons for heavy periods are greatly varied. A physical cause will be discovered in many cases. Fibroids can cause excessive blood loss, but so too can tiny polyps (no more significant perhaps than a nasal polyp). But medical opinion must always be sought without delay. Upsets of the endocrine secretions of the body are often implicated. Sometimes the lining of the womb just seems to get shed irregularly, and so the uterus cannot contract normally and thus stop bleeding at the end of a period.

Heavy periods in young women can occur when they opt for intra-uterine device (IUD) contraceptive practice. In older women, menorrhagia can be a sign of approaching menopause, and if it is severe enough, is the commonest reason for the operation of hysterectomy. Persistent menorrhagia, whether in young or pre-menopausal women, should always warrant a thorough search for gynaecological abnormality.

Orthodox Medical Management

Heavy periods are very common, especially at puberty or at the end of menstrual life, but anything out of the ordinary is a signal for seeking medical advice. Internal examination while actually menstruating is possible if this is absolutely necessary, but it is best to wait for the period to have stopped for a few days before an examination. This is the only delay that should be countenanced.

No one can tell the cause of a particular menorrhagia until after investigation. If the uterus is found to be healthy, the reason is probably hormonal imbalance, and sometimes supplementation of a progestogen is given; sometimes the progestogen-only contraceptive pill can help as well (although there are risks of side effects).

Good Health-Food Management

VITAMIN E AND IUD MENORRHAGIA

The effectiveness of Vitamin E is cited in the *Nutritional Desk Reference*, by R.H. Garrison and E. Somer (Keats Publishing, 1985).

A group of 51 women suffering from IUD-type menorrhagia were treated with Vitamin E in a dose of 100mg every other day. In practically every participant the monthly blood loss fell to pre-IUD levels.

IRON AND MENORRHAGIA

Menorrhagia in healthy young women in whom gynaecological abnormality has been excluded may benefit from iron supplementation. Such women may not be 'anaemic' in as much as their haemoglobin levels (the usual yardstick of a diagnosis of anaemia) are normal. If, however, their *serum iron* is measured it is sometimes found to be lowered. Iron supplementation seems to be particularly enhanced in such cases by co-supplements of Vitamin C. (Dyspepsia may occur as a side effect in all iron medication.)

Many older menorrhagic patients respond to supplementation of their diet with adequate iron preparations – ferrous sulphate or ferrous gluconate, 600mg daily – and as their serum iron improves so do their symptoms. In one double blind study, 75 per cent of menorrhagic older patients improved on iron supplementation compared with 32.5 per cent taking placebo – a significant difference. This must have been one of the best-kept secrets of medical gynaecology!

It would seem that many women who experience heavy periods are poor iron absorbers.

GOOD BUYS

- Vitamin E • Iron/vitamin complexes.

See also: **Dysmenorrhoea; Menopausal Problems and Iron; Vitamins C and E.**

MIGRAINE

Migraine means recurrent headaches associated with visual and gastrointestinal upset, and about 10 per cent of the population suffer to some extent. The cause of migraine is unknown, although the pain is said to be related to unexplained widening and narrowing of blood vessels in the head. The headache is often throbbing and one-sided. Sometimes there is a tingling sensation in the limbs, together with a transient weakness. Prior to a migraine attack, suffers sometimes experience a feeling of well-being. Visual symptoms – partial loss of vision, flashes of light, or zig-zag lines – are 'seen', then in a quarter of an hour or so, the headache comes on, nausea increases, sometimes followed by vomiting, and sufferers seek out a darkened room in which to lie down.

Alcohol and certain foods such as chocolate and cheese are often implicated in migraine attacks. They contain a substance to which blood vessels are sensitive.

Orthodox Medical Management

For the actual attack painkillers (such as paracetamol) and anti-sickness drugs (Metoclopramide) are prescribed with or without an ergotomine drug (one that constricts small blood vessels and stimulates the endings of the sympathetic nerves). Because medical treatment is often less than effective, doctors have sought out several prophylactic (preventative) remedies, including Pizotifen, Propranolol, Clonidine and Methysergide. All have significant side effects.

Good Health-Food Management

Quite recently a herbal remedy, *Tanacetum parthenium*, or the herbal plant feverfew, has proved itself to be a Gold Standard prophylactic remedy for migraine in two well-designed, double blinded trails carried out at medical centres of excellence. Patients taking capsules containing 25mg of dried feverfew leaf twice daily experienced fewer attacks and a reduction of severity of attacks. See Herbalist Products.

There appear to be few adverse side effects of feverfew in this dosage, and no contraindications of its use.

GOOD BUYS

★ Gold Standard
● Feverfew preparations in 25mg doses (LIFEPLAN or HEALTHCRAFTS).

See also: **Herbalist Products (Feverfew).**

MULTIPLE SCLEROSIS (MS)

Considerable personal soul-searching preceded the decision to include any reference to this miserable disease of unknown origin in a book on health foods. This is because there is no justification for making *any* claim for therapy, either at an orthodox or any other level, that really stands up to a bold critical analysis. One does, however, come across patients who feel so totally convinced they have been helped by a type of health food therapy that it seems inhumane, in a way, not to mention this in a book which aims to give a wider knowledge of health foods and their potential benefits.

MS is an incurable disease of the nervous system in which the protective myelin sheaths covering the nerves of the body become inflamed and eventually degenerate so much that sufferers can sometimes become severely disabled. Depending on where the disease strikes, the occurrence of symptoms can vary, and there is commonly a pattern of relapses and remissions. Some sufferers have an initial attack and diagnosis, then remain symptom-free for many years.

MS initially manifests mostly between the ages of 25 and 35.

In the UK alone there are about 50,000 sufferers. Strangely, its incidence is related to the distance lived from the equator: at 50–60°N the incidence is 60–100 per 100,000 people; in latitudes below 30°N the prevalence is fewer than 10 per 100,000 inhabitants. In the southern hemisphere the incidence is very similarly related to the distance lived from the equator. Most data suggests that MS is an acquired environmental disease that occurs in a genetically susceptible host (first-degree relatives of an existing MS sufferer have an above-average incidence of MS), and that a 'window' of susceptibility for infection occurs at around puberty.

Signs and Symptoms

These depend upon the sites at which MS strikes. The optic nerves can be affected, with mild eye pain and blurring of vision leading to severe but usually temporary visual loss. Any loss of power or sensation in limbs should be investigated, as should any signs of ataxia (uncoordination of muscular action usually without loss of muscular power) or persistent vertigo (giddiness), because MS can disclose itself in such symptoms.

Orthodox Medical and Good Health-Food Management

Diet has often played a large part in orthodox treatment. Gluten, for instance, has sometimes been omitted from the diet.

Perhaps the most interesting postulate is that a high intake of saturated fats in the diet should be avoided in MS. In Norway, where this has been evaluated, there is a low incidence of MS in coastal fishing areas compared with agricultural communities in the same latitudes.

One of the great difficulties is that in MS, once the damage has been done to the nerves involved in the MS process, then it is probably too late to put matters right by means of dietary intervention. But in one experimental study involving 146 patients who were placed on a low-fat diet for 17 years, it was demonstrated that the disease was less rapidly progressive than it was in matched untreated cases. What is more, if treatment was initiated very early on in the illness a high percentage of patients remained unchanged for up to 20 years. Patients who replaced their saturated fat intake with more polyunsaturated fats in the diet also deteriorated the least during the period.

Several published trials of very variable design and analysis have looked quite critically at the polyunsaturated fatty acids with reference to the progression of the disease. A review article in the *Lancet* looked at three double blind trials of linoleic acid in MS patients who were suffering from a typical remitting-relapsing type of illness. It involved 87 treated patients and controls. The interesting thing was that patients who entered the trial with minimal disability fared better on therapy than did more handicapped controls and they experienced smaller increases of disability than did such controls.

Long-term supplementation of the diet with EFA-rich polyunsaturated oils seems to be most beneficial to the MS victim, mainly, if not entirely, in the context of reducing episodes of degenerative disease and prolonging remissions. One study suggests that really long periods of treatment, in excess of two years, are indicated if myelin protection against MS is to be fostered.

There is, of course, a 'Catch 22' situation with reference to trials centred on improved remissions of this baffling disease, for one can only *guess* at what the remission profile is liable to be in the absence of *any* treatment schedule. Nevertheless, if a treatment system is non-toxic, non-invasive, and has other positive health connotations, then it would seem only reasonable to give it a full and prolonged trial in MS victims.

GOOD BUYS

● MAXEPA (NOVEX) and linoleic acid products seem to qualify.

Rich sources of linoleic acid include corn oil and many other vegetable oils. A tablespoon daily of corn, safflower or sunflower oil would provide adequate dietary enrichment.

See also: **Cod Liver Oil; Glossary; Marine Oils; Plant Oils.**

OSTEOPOROSIS

OSTEORPOROSIS is an age-related disorder of the bone, characterised by decreased bone mass and by an increased susceptibility to fractures which occur in the absence of any obvious cause. The Office of Medical Applications of Research in Bethesda, Maryland, states that in the USA alone there are 15–20 million sufferers, and the disorder causes about 1.3 million fractures each year. In the UK there are probably 1.7 million sufferers, mostly over the age of 45. If you are lucky enough to reach the age of 90, there is a 32 per cent chance of your suffering from an osteoporotic hip fracture if you are a woman and a 12 per cent chance if you are a man. In other words, osteoporosis is a very common disease of the elderly and a great charge on the NHS and medical services the world over.

To understand a little better about osteoporosis you have to know a little more about bone. Bone is basically a gelatinous tissue that is intimately impregnated with minerals, notably calcium and phosphorus, but also with magnesium. It is a mistake to think of bone as an inanimate sort of tissue, as it in fact undergoes a continuous remodelling (turnover) all through life, and is very much alive. Cells called osteoclasts constantly reabsorb bone while other cells called osteoblasts re-form bone. Normally bone reabsorption and formation are linked closely, and all sorts of factors, including mechanical and nutritional forces and hormone levels, influence the remodelling process.

We all reach our peak bone mass at the age of about 35, but sex, race, nutritional profile, exercise habits and overall health all influence peak bone massing to a variable extent. In men the total mass of bone at its peak is 30 per cent more than it is in women. There is an interesting racial variation too, for bone mass is about 10 per cent higher in black people than it is in white.

After reaching its peak, your bone mass starts to decline due to an imbalance of the modelling process, and then bones gradually start to lose both their mineral and their gelatinous matrix. But they still retain their basic organisation and function quite well if given the chance. In women the menopause, or change of life, brings a sort of crisis in bone remodelling which lasts for between three and seven years, during which a rapid decrease of bone mass occurs. Because of the sudden hormone depletion at this time, women sustain more osteoporosis fractures in the post-menopausal years. Hormone replacement therapy (HRT) can call a partial halt to this decline in women.

To some extent the progression down the road of disability seems to have been accepted by the medical profession as being inevitable once an osteoporosis fracture has occurred. Sadly, most patients with hip fractures fail to recover their previous degree of activity, and nearly 20 per cent die during the following year. Fractures involving the vertebrae (bones of the backbone), wrist and arms are often the starting point of loss of confidence, loss of mobility and a general decline unless everybody works hard to prevent this state of affairs.

Signs and Symptoms

In most cases osteoporosis is symptomless until complications occur. But not always. If osteoporotic bones get compressed in your neck or back region, odd aches and pains follow and you may finish up wearing a neck collar or a bracing corset.

Unfortunately, too, there is no quick and easy diagnostic test for osteoporosis. Even X-rays that normally tell us so much about bone will only clinch a diagnosis when there is an advanced progress of the disease with a loss of 30 – 50 per cent of skeletal mass. This being so, earlier diagnosis must rest on a high level of suspicion – much higher than is prevalent generally today – both by you and your doctor. All over-50s have a degree of osteoporosis and the trick is to keep it at bay. Prophylaxis is much more effective than treatment as, once lost, bone mass cannot be restored.

Orthodox Medical and Good Health-Food Management

Clearly, special-risk groups should be very carefully monitored and energetically treated (for example, women at the menopause, those who have had hysterectomy operations – particularly those in which the ovaries are removed as well as the womb – or who have suffered from a premature menopause). It has been proved without doubt that the female sex hormone oestrogen allows women to retain more of their mineral intake, but this facility disappears at the menopause. The reason that there is a later peak in osteoporosis problems in men than in women seems to be due to the fact that, hormonally at least, men remain 'sexual' for much longer than women do, producing testosterone, the male sex hormone, well into old age.

The common clinical symptoms of osteoporosis should no longer be ignored by doctors and patients alike. The general shrinking of the skeleton, the 'buffalo' hump at the base of the neck, the aches and pains in hands and arms brought about by compression effects on nerves as they leave the spinal cord for the arms, together with the observation that 'Grandma is growing downwards' are too often ignored. Such symptoms tend to be shrugged off as part of the decline of advancing years.

This attitude was understandable perhaps when, generally speaking, specific treatment for osteoporosis was unsatisfactory (apart from hormone replacement therapy in menopausal women). But today, when it has been proved that good health-food supplements improve bone strength and mineral retention, the nasty, crippling disease of osteoporosis must surely be acknowledged as being preventable.

CALCIUM AND OSTEOPOROSIS

For years now physicians have paid lip service to the principle of the dietary management of osteoporosis, but in a Consensus Conference on osteoporosis published in the *New England Journal of Medicine* in 1993 there is up-to-date endorsement of the view which advocates increasing calcium intake to 1,000mg per day to combat the disease, and some authorities recommend 1,500mg after the menopause.

On average the intake of calcium is much lower than the RNI of 700mg per day, so supplementation is advisable and can be very helpful.

However, many foods affect the utilisation of calcium – phosphates, oxalates (green vegetables) and phytates – and so dietary calcium has to be carefully considered in relation to other nutrients. A high-calcium diet may not necessarily protect against osteoporosis if the diet is equally high in phosphates: foods which contain more phosphates than calcium include meat, poultry and fish, for example.

A deficiency of Vitamin D adversely affects the absorption of calcium, so adequate Vitamin D intake should be maintained. Also, because calcium and magnesium compete for intestinal absorption, there is a case for taking extra magnesium as well.

MAGNESIUM AND OSTEOPOROSIS

Very slowly it is being realised that magnesium can also make an important contribution to osteoporosis prophylaxis. Relatively little attention has been paid to the importance of magnesium in bone metabolism, other than the fact that it clearly influences the activity of the parathyroid glands. These tiny structures in the neck are very closely linked to the mechanism of bone mineralisation.

One of the reasons that doctors, generally speaking, are not over-enthusiastic about considering magnesium deficiency as a cause for many of our ills is because routine blood tests for magnesium are usually constant. But blood tests do not disclose abnormality of magnesium in the *tissues*. For blood magnesium does not go up and down in magnesium tissue deficiency as, for instance, does iron in the blood when the body becomes anaemic. Plasma levels of magnesium are automatically maintained within very narrow limits from magnesium stores, even in the face of insufficiency of magnesium intake or excessive losses. The major depot of stored magnesium is our bones which contain two-thirds of our total body magnesium: if the body's magnesium is mobilised from tissue stores in cases of magnesium imbalance then bones must become less healthy – or at least quite different in their mineral content.

In young animals this bone-bound magnesium is relatively labile (prone to chemical change) and easily mobilised. No doubt in young people this plays a large part in keeping magnesium levels in the body stable. But as age increases, and especially if low magnesium intake persists, and if absorption is poor or dietary factors exist that compete for magnesium, then as tissue magnesium falls, disturbances of bone modelling slowly and inevitably occur.

A high calcium intake may not be all that effective all the time in combating osteoporosis because it competes with magnesium for intestinal absorption. Excess of phosphate in the diet also decreases vital bone magnesium, too.

VITAMIN D AND OSTEOPOROSIS

Because of its relationship with the mineral calcium – promoting its absorption, and therefore the mineralisation of bones – Vitamin D has become increasingly valued in the management of the brittle bones of osteoporosis.

GOOD BUYS

● For the magnesium factor in osteoporosis, Magnesium-OK (WASSEN) ● For calcium supplementation: Calcia (ENGLISH GRAINS HEALTHCARE); Extra Calcium (BIO HEALTH); Aminochel Calcium (HEALTHCRAFTS) ● Vitamin D supplements (see page 143).

See also: **Ageing; Menopausal Problems; Calcium; Magnesium; Vitamin D.**

PERIODONTAL DISEASE

THIS is a term applied to a disease of the mouth, primarily of the gums. It was once called gingivitis (inflammation of the gingival margins, or gums) and pyorrhoea (relating to the dischange of pus, a sign of advanced gum disease). The disease attacks the gum where it meets the tooth, and can lead to teeth loosening in the jaw, and ultimately falling out. All too often the only effective treatment the dentist can offer is extraction and subsequent dentures.

Energetic research has led to a vast improvement in the management of periodontal disease, and it is now widely accepted that both dental decay (dental caries) and the gingivitis that signals periodontal disease are related to plaque. Plaque is a gelatinous deposit which adheres firmly to teeth and separates them from the gum tissues. It is composed of a dense mass of micro-organisms of many and varied kinds growing within a matrix of sugary substances (polysaccharides). These micro-organisms produce toxins which attack the gums and the specialised periodontal fibres which attach the teeth to the bony jaw. Eventually, if unchecked, the tooth enamel is also attacked; some severe forms of the disease can actually eat into the bone of the jaw itself.

Signs and Symptoms

The earliest signs of dental caries will probably only be noticed by the dentist, but you can spot incipient gum disease yourself at home. Any bleeding from the gums when you brush your teeth is a sign that the gums are under threat of disease. The next symptoms are swollen red gums with some tenderness, bad breath, and there may be a bad taste in the mouth. If the gums are receding (this is a natural ageing process, and why we become 'long in the tooth'), or there is a change of bite or in fit of dentures, the mouth geography may be altering and disease is taking hold. At the very first sign of blood during tooth cleaning, the dentist should be consulted if the disease is to be halted and teeth are to be saved.

Orthodox Dental Management

Prevention of periodontal disease is best accomplished by a partnership in dental hygiene embarked upon by the dentist and the patient. Regular and careful tooth cleaning, the use of dental floss and toothpicks backed up by suitable anti-caries and anti-plaque toothpastes and plaque-disclosing techniques, should accompany six-monthly dental inspections and, if necessary, tooth scaling. This latter is a procedure needed for the removal of tartar or plaque. Scaling can only be performed by the dentist or dental hygienist.

Good Health-Food Management

Until comparatively recently, if you could not afford regular prophylactic dentistry or had phobic fears of dental treatment, you could only rely on such aids to dental hygiene as were available in the previously mentioned procedures and products. But there are several health foods that are relevant to mouth health, and many nutritionists and dentists believe *diet* is a major influence on the health of the teeth and gums. Sugar is the well-known enemy (the plaque bacteria flourish in a sugary environment), but a good balanced diet, perhaps supplemented by health foods, is as important to the continuing health of the teeth as it is to the rest of the body.

VITAMIN C AND PERIODONTAL DISEASE

Vitamin C is particularly necessary for the health of all connective tissue, and there is no connective tissue more vital to our well-being than that which binds our teeth to our jaws. It is one of the odd quirks of Nature that certain groups of animals (which include humankind, our fellow primates and, strangely, guinea pigs) lack a specialised enzyme system that converts glucose into Vitamin C. Because we cannot make or store Vitamin C in the body to any extent (see page 134), to preserve dental and periodontal health we need adequate daily Vitamin C intake, in the form of fruit or supplement.

Vitamin C's relationship with gum health is often forgotten, although it has long been established. In scurvy, an early sign is bleeding gums: at this stage small haemorrhages are occurring in the connective tissues that bind our teeth and jaws together, and so gingivitis is manifest. Many holistic dentists use large doses of Vitamin C to slow down the progress of gum disease.

CALCIUM AND PERIODONTAL DISEASE

Calcium has as vital a relationship to mouth health as does Vitamin C. Adequate calcification of the teeth is very important at particular times in the life of a tooth – during pregnancy, when the baby's teeth are being formed, and when the adult teeth are being formed in a child, up to about 12 years old, and so at this time adequate calcium intake is vital. A good diet, with plenty of calcium foods, is particularly necessary when the baby is in the womb; this is primarily to help the mother, for the needs of the baby have priority, and she may suffer calcium loss from her bones. In the past, mothers feared 'losing a tooth for each baby'. This was probably due to periodontal disease.

FLUORIDE AND PERIODONTAL DISEASE

On the whole, fluoride is looked upon as a dental saviour when it is used to prevent dental caries developing. It does this by forming a sort of coating on the teeth; it also interferes with the growth of bacterial plaques, and modifies the acids they produce (which is what eats into the enamel). However, many people worry about the concentrations of fluoride: 1 part per million is safe, but even a fraction above that can affect the teeth, and fluorosis – or a coloured mottling of the teeth – can result. Children are particularly vulnerable in that they could be drinking fluoridated water and they could be ingesting more fluoride from their toothpaste.

COENZYME Q10 AND PERIODONTAL DISEASE

In 1976 it was suggested that a substance known as Coenzyme Q10 (CoQ10) may be deficient in cases of periodontal disease.

As a result, two experimental double blind studies showed that CoQ10 in doses of 50mg per day resulted in a significant improvement of gingival health compared with the placebo substance administered in the trial. Although relatively small in total numbers of patients involved, these trials led to an article in a reputable publication, *Chemical and Clinical Pharmacology*, assessing seven studies which reviewed over 300 patients, 70 per cent of whom responded favourably to CoQ10. The dental surgeons who were involved with these studies were clearly very impressed with the therapy.

GOOD BUYS

★ *Gold Standard*
• Coenzyme Q10 (HEALTHILIFE and WASSEN).

Useful
• Vitamin C preparations   • Calcium preparations.

Worth Trying
• Anti-plaque preparations available in the pharmacy.

See also: **Calcium; Coenzyme Q10; Fluoride; Vitamin C.**

PMS OR PRE-MENSTRUAL SYNDROME

THE pre-menstrual sydrome is a unique condition, for it was more or less discovered by a French criminologist over 100 years ago who noted that 63 per cent of all women apprehended for shoplifting were in a pre-menstrual phase of their monthly cycle. But it was not until 1931 that doctors became interested when a US gynaecologist called Robert Frank described a series of 15 women who suffered from a syndrome that involved irritability, anxiety, depression and a feeling of being blown up or bloated in the days before they menstruated, or during the first four days of the menstrual flow.

Today we define PMS as the occurrence of a variety of apparently unrelated symptoms that are seen only in the second half of the menstrual cycle and which disappear during the early days of the menstrual period.

PMS is also referred to as PMT, or pre-menstrual tension. Between 20 and 30 per cent of women experience PMS at some time.

Arguments about the fundamental cause of PMS have preoccupied research workers for years. Because of the cyclical nature of the problem, clinical trials have been difficult to design and interpret. Many of the classic symptoms of PMS are difficult to quantify, too. For instance, how do you measure a feeling of being bloated or irritable? Double blind trials, in which nobody (that is, neither doctor nor patient) knows who is receiving a drug under test for evaluation and who is receiving a dummy placebo tablet, have been difficult to design and to recruit.

PMS is well-recognised for its facility to trigger off psychological problems. For instance, women who are known to suffer episodes of psychiatric illness are much more likely to relapse or be admitted into hospital because of these conditions during the pre-menstrual days of their lives than at other times.

It also seems true that women who are psychiatrically ill suffer PMS more severely than do fitter women.

Signs and Symptoms

Some would say that PMS has no specific symptomatology and that any symptoms of a *cyclical* nature related to menstruation 'diagnose' the disease. Indeed, before making a diagnosis of PMS many doctors ask patients to keep a diary in which they note from day to day the symptoms that are worrying. Often this alone is substantially therapeutic, as sufferers come to accept the true nature of their problem. Relief that they are neither going mad nor suffering from some alarming and incurable disease understandably brings everything into a healthier perspective.

Two degrees of PMS occur. About 90 per cent of women experience a mild form lasting three to four days. More severe cases suffer quite different and unpleasant symptoms which may last from seven to fourteen days before the period starts. Distress is often severe enough to disrupt family and working relationships, and to curtail normal activities.

A 'syndrome' is just the medical jargon for a collection of symptoms, and there are several predominant types of PMS.

ANXIETY-DOMINATED PMS

In this condition, all the common manifestations of anxiety seem to 'home in' on the victim at period times in an accentuated manner and tax her coping mechanisms unduly. Symptoms include palpitations, sweating, urinary frequency, dizziness, headache, poor appetite, strange and inexplicable abdominal cramps, a tendency for the hands and fingers to shake inexplicably, sleeplessness or excessive tiredness and panic states. What spouses, friends and children call 'impossible behaviour' is commonplace in this sort of PMS. Alongside these and other symptoms, in some anxiety-dominated PMS victims, a distinct tendency is to consume excessive quantities of dairy produce and/or refined sugars.

Anxiety-dominated PMS is characterised biochemically by

elevated levels of blood oestrogen and a low blood progesterone, and so it is the most likely type of PMS to respond to medical treatment with progesterone (see Glossary).

DEPRESSION-DOMINATED PMS

This is the most potentially worrying type of PMS, for there is a well-documented peak incidence of suicide in the pre-menstrual days, and depression is a subject that cries out for prompt and effective medical treatment at all times. It is extremely difficult for even a trained medical or psychiatric observer to gauge the 'depth' of a depressed state, and, for lay workers, management of depressive illness is fraught with hazard. PMS victims in whom apathy, loss of attention to dress, make-up or general appearance, crying, withdrawal, forgetfulness or confusion manifest should be treated in the doctor's consulting room and not at the health-food shop.

PMS-H

This is shorthand jargon for what is sometimes called hyperhydration PMS, in which there is a feeling of bloatedness, excessive breast tenderness, or a sudden weight gain of over 1.4kg (3lb) during the pre-menstrual time. To some extent, water and salt retention (causing body bloating) is part and parcel of all PMS, but in PMS-H this is predominant.

Orthodox Medical Management

The most fashionable theory for PMS today is that the disease is due to some imbalance between the two sex hormones, progesterone and oestrogen, which, by means of a very neat biological ebb and flow system, control and regulate the whole process of ovulation (egg cell release) and regulate menstruation. The previously-held 'hormone theory' for PMS – that it was simply due to lack of one hormone, progesterone – is no longer so tenable because many investigations of PMS victims have disclosed normal progesterone levels even in severe sufferers. Nevertheless, giving extra progesterone does seem to help certain PMS victims, probably because this has some effect on the centres that regulate the whole intricate system of female sex biochemistry.

However, it is not universally effective, and side effects can cause problems. It is not recommended in women who have suffered thrombosis disorder or those who suffer undiagnosed vaginal bleeding or liver disease.

Good Health-Food Management

There is a curious reluctance in doctors to accept that anything other than hormone manipulation is 'proper' treatment of PMS. This is despite the publication of several well-designed trials, the most impressive of which are published in medical journals of high repute and authority, which indicate that health food manipulation has a part to play in the management of this wretched condition.

EVENING PRIMROSE OIL AND PMS

There is increasing evidence – from both sufferers and manufacturers – that a daily dose of evening primrose oil can benefit PMS, whether banishing symptoms altogether, or by preventing the bloatedness and breast pain of periods.

Between four and eight capsules should be taken during the two weeks that precede a period, and this may be combined with a mineral supplement, the most logical of which would be Magnesium-OK.

GINSENG AND PMS

The anxiety-relieving qualities of ginseng could well help the anxiety-dominated PMS. Ginseng has a reputation for the enhancement of the ability to cope with stress, and PMS victims are often very stress-ridden with their miserable disability.

MAGNESIUM AND PMS

A slight variation of anxiety-dominated PMS is sometimes referred to as PMS-C, in which a craving for sweet things is prevalent during the pre-menstrual days, as well as headache, palpitations, fainting attacks and abnormal fatigue. At this time, a low red-cell magnesium level has been reported in such women, and this type of PMS may well respond to magnesium supplementation.

VITAMIN B$_6$ AND PMS

Anxiety-dominated PMS responds favourably sometimes to Vitamin B$_6$ (pyridoxine).

There are complex hormonal causes for the symptoms of PMS-H – the bloating form of PMS – but these can sometimes be relieved by Vitamin B$_6$ therapy.

VITAMIN E AND PMS

Vitamin E has been found to be particularly useful in relieving the breast tenderness in PMS-H, especially if Vitamin E is combined with a low-sodium diet.

GOOD BUYS

● Efamol Pre-Menstrual Pack (BRITANNIA HEALTH).

Useful for anxiety-dominated PMS
● Magnesium-OK (WASSEN) contains Vitamin E, magnesium and pyridoxine.

Worth Trying (for anxiety-dominated PMS)
● Ginseng.

Useful (for PMS-H)
● Vitamins E + B$_6$.

See also: **Evening Primrose Oil; Ginseng; Magnesium; Plant Oils; Vitamins B$_6$ and E and Dysmenorrhoea; Menorrhagia; Tension and Stress; Tiredness and Fatigue.**

POOR CIRCULATION (CHILBLAINS)

ONE of the functions of the circulation is to regulate the body temperature by altering the blood flow through the skin. This is done by nervous impulses stimulating the muscular walls of the arterial vessels to contract or relax. Various chemical substances in the blood can act directly on these tiny muscular structures.

Strangely, there is a curious 'sexism' about this regulatory system. Men tend to maintain their skin vessels in a state of 'open all hours' (and, incidentally, lose over 10 per cent of their body heat through their skin all the time as a result). Women seem to function more conservatively, opening up or shutting down skin circulation much more than do men. This is probably why women complain of 'poor circulation' more than men, and suffer from a variety of circulatory problems that in medical textbooks earn such important-sounding names as *Raynaud's phenomenon, erythromelagia, erythrocyanosis* and *acrocyanosis*. The most prevalent is *chilblains*, which doctors call *pernio*.

Signs and Symptoms

Blanched or blue areas occur on the fingers, toes, ears, feet or, more rarely, on cheeks and nose. If rubbed, or when they are getting warm, these areas go red and itch and burn. Sometimes swelling and blistering occurs. Fingers and legs feel cold to the touch.

Orthodox Medical Management

Doctors have really been quite unsuccessful in devising effective remedies for poor circulation problems. But this has not prevented them prescribing many drugs called vasodilators, although there is little evidence that stands up to Gold Standard appraisal on this score.

Happily, surgeons have largely abandoned tricky operations aimed at improving poor circulation that were once quite popular too. Most doctors simply advise the wearing of warm and waterproof clothing and plenty of outdoor exercise.

Good Health-Food Management

Although to a large extent poor circulation problems are best coped with by means of common-sense wrapping up, and avoiding damp-cold, the possibilities of health-food aid should not be ignored.

VITAMIN B₃ AND POOR CIRCULATION

Large doses of Vitamin B_3 (niacin or nicotinic acid) cause the skin to flush, therefore galvanising the circulation into action, and this has proved particularly useful in chilblain sufferers.

GOOD BUYS

• Yeast is a popular health-food source of Vitamin B_3. The practice of taking yeast tablets for the circulation would seemed to be backed with evidence that it 'works' as well as, and possibly better than, some prescription remedies. Large and conclusive medical trials are unlikely because of the non-patentability of yeast • But some would argue that Vitamin B_3 (when taken as niacin tablets in doses from 25 – 100mg), which has a vasodilator effect of about 2 hours duration, and may be associated with some itching and burning especially evident in the 'blush' area, is more scientific than yeast and therefore better • Some multivitamin tablets contain meaningful amounts of Vitamin B_3. There are over 30 products on offer at most health food outlets, and availability and price dictates the best buy.

See also: Vitamin B_3.

PROSTATITIS AND PROSTATE PROBLEMS

PROSTATITIS is an imperfectly understood condition that is probably the result of inflammation of the prostate gland, a fibro-muscular structure that encircles the base of the bladder in the sexually mature male.

Signs and Symptoms

Prostatitis announces its presence in various ways. Sometimes the victim experiences a 'flu-like illness associated with difficulty in urination in which symptoms of urgency to pass urine, painful urination or urinary retention may occur. This acute form of prostatitis may respond to medical treatment with antibiotics or it may proceed to a more chronic condition of bladder irritation in which painful urination, frequency of urination, difficulty in starting urination, a necessity to pass urine at night and a urethral discharge are the presenting symptoms and signs.

At this stage there is a considerable overlap with the condition known as *prostatism*, so far as symptoms are concerned. Prostatism is brought about by an over-growth of the fibro-muscular and glandular substance of the prostate gland, and the clinical manifestations of this condition include urinary hesitancy and frequency, a decreased flow and force of the urinary stream, a necessity to pass urine during the night, urgency of micturation and sometimes acute retention of urine.

Orthodox Medical Management

So far as prostatitis is concerned, antibiotics are the mainstay of treatment. Once prostate gland over-growth (hyperplasia) has developed, an operation (prostatectomy) is necessary, and more than 50,000 prostatectomies are performed in the UK each year (300,000 in the USA). Two types of operation are available: the 'open' prostatectomy, so-called because it involves an incision to open the abdomen and bladder, and the transurethral prostatectomy in which the prostate is 'tunnelled' out by means of an instrument that is passed up through the penis.

Good Health-Food Management

Recently medical trials have shown that a particular type of rye grass pollen extract, known as Cernilton, is effective in the management of chronic prostatitis, provided complicating factors (urethral stricture, urinary stone or bladder neck narrowing) are absent.

Another double blind, placebo-controlled study of 60 patients with urinary problems due to prostatic hypertrophy showed that there was a statistically significant improvement in the symptomatology of 69 per cent of patients taking Cernilton compared with 30 per cent of patients taking a placebo.

GOOD BUYS

★ *Gold Standard*
● Cernilton, marketed in the UK as Prostabrit (BRITANNIA HEALTH): 2 tablets with water first thing in the morning or at night.

See also: **Pollen, Propolis and Royal Jelly.**

RICKETS

RICKETS is a curious disease that baffled doctors for years, because it could be cured and prevented in two different ways – either by sunshine, or by a diet that contained adequate Vitamin D. This vitamin is necessary for the absorption and use of the mineral calcium in the body. If there is a lack of it, bone deformity – the 'bandy legs' of rickets – can result.

Your skin can produce its own Vitamin D providing it is exposed regularly to adequate doses of sunshine. But cases of rickets are still reported in Europe and elsewhere from time to time in immigrants, coloured people used to sunnier climes, who wrap up well in the colder, less sunny weather. Poor diet also plays a part. In dark and smoky mid-17th-century industrial Britain, rickets was so prevalent that it was called the 'English Disease', and until the turn of the century it plagued the poverty-stricken communities in many parts of the country, due to a combination of lack of exposure to sunshine and lack of Vitamin D-rich produce. Third World countries still suffer the disease.

Orthodox Medical Management

During the Second World War, egg and fat rationing placed the UK population at wholesale risk of rickets because these foods are important natural Vitamin D sources. But an epidemic of rickets in children did not develop because cod liver oil was freely available for babies and toddlers.

Good Health-Food Management

Unless dairy produce and fish are eaten as a regular part of everyday nutrition, or the climate offers a fair exposure to sunlight, many people still live on a diet which is on the borderline as far as rickets is concerned. Cod liver oil and Vitamin D supplementation is the answer.

GOOD BUYS

★ *Gold Standard*
● All cod liver oil products.

See also: **Cod Liver Oil; Marine Oils; Vitamin D.**

TENSION AND STRESS

TENSION and stress are part of everyday existence. Often they have helpful and productive functions – as a spur to peaks of performance we could not otherwise reach. But chronic tension and stress can have a darker side, and erupt as disabling anxiety and depression. Even the most sophisticated psychotherapists have difficulty in defining the *ultimate* cause of anxiety, tension and stress symptoms. Some argue that they are the result of disturbed awareness in an 'inadequate' or 'immature' personality.

An odd characteristic of tension and stress symptoms is that they are often *organ-specific* – in other words, they produce gut symptomatology (IBS), or cardiac symptoms (palpitations), or sexual symptoms (erection failure, or dyspareunia).

The signs and symptoms are so various that it would be impossible to list them here, but many of the illnesses and diseases throughout this book can be related to or caused by stress and tension.

Orthodox Medical Management

Medicine today has a broad spectrum of psychoactive drugs. Hypnotics and sedatives like diazepam (Valium) compounds are highly effective in damping down some of the symptoms of anxiety. But often there is unpleasant 'rebound' anxiety as the drug effect wears off, and so habituation problems often occur with these drugs. Social stimulants like the caffeine in tea and coffee are, of course, widely used. The amphetamine drugs (benzedrine), although effective for short-term use to combat stress, fatigue and exhaustion, are potentially addictive, and capable of producing wild behaviour and withdrawal symptoms. They too are bedevilled with other side effects.

Good Health-Food Management

I must admit that evidence for health-food benefit is slim in many cases, but health foods may well help in certain circumstances and are supported by some scientific evidence. Anything that is non-toxic, non-addictive and which might just ameliorate some of the symptoms of stress is worth trying.

GINSENG AND TENSION AND STRESS

The attraction of using ginseng psychotrophically is that it appears to be a substance that allows the body to *adapt* to stress. The very term *adaptogen* (see below) is an apt one, for ginseng does not produce much in the way of feelings of over-excitation and, if taken in reasonable doses, it does not disturb sleep patterns in the same way as other psychotrophics.

To understand the adaptogen principle one has to consider the development of 'coping skills' which allow us to face up to, and tolerate, various levels of anxiety in everyday life. Much of modern stress management is a practical exercise in the development of these coping skills, without which people often appear to be incapacitated by their experience of anxiety. Part of ginseng's therapeutic spectrum would seem to be a pharmacological *enhancement* of nature's facility to develop coping skills, which allow the often heavily-disabled anxious person to behave more logically and more normally.

ZINC AND TENSION AND STRESS

There is considerable evidence that zinc supplementation can help in many diseases which are associated with emotional and physical stress – the acne which appears in a pubertal boy, the bulimia or anorexia which develops in a teenage girl. In both of these miserable, stress-related diseases, zinc supplements have proved to be useful.

HERBALIST PRODUCTS AND TENSION AND STRESS

Although many herbal remedies are largely unproven in any scientific sense, there are several products which have been selling successfully for many years. Others have a proven pharmacological action.

GOOD BUYS

★ *Gold Standard*
● Zinc preparations.

Useful
● Ginseng ● Herbalist products.

See also: **Acne; Anorexia Nervosa; Cardiac Problems: Hypertension; Insomnia; Irritable Bowel Syndrome; Ginseng; Herbalist Products; Zinc.**

TIREDNESS AND FATIGUE

CHRONIC tiredness and fatigue are extremely common. A recent Royal College of General Practitioners' survey pointed out that 24 patients in every practice felt bad enough on this score to see their GP every year and another 150 described it as a secondary symptom. In many ways this problem is an 'iceberg' symptom: if people keep symptom diaries, 'tired all the time' crops up extremely frequently.

Signs and Symptoms

These need no explanation. Whether or not a particular post-viral 'tired all the time' syndrome exists is still a matter for medical debate.

Orthodox Medical Management

Sufferers often get scant attention from their doctors, largely because even batteries of sophisticated tests disclose no convincing abnormalities. The diagnosis of 'neurosis' is never far from most doctors' lips in such cases.

Good Health-Food Management

It would be great if it were possible to instantly and universally combat general tiredness and fatigue by means of a health-food product. But many would argue that this would only be likely if the health food in question treats an *overt* nutritional deficiency that has persisted for some time. On occasion, of course, a deficiency state relative to a particular vitamin, say, can be present and cause symptoms. It seems likely that quite pronounced long-term nutritional deficiencies are necessary before tiredness and fatigue symptoms erupt.

291

VITAMINS, TIREDNESS AND FATIGUE

Nevertheless, it has been demonstrated, for instance, that if the recommended allowance of the B complex vitamins is decreased by 45 per cent then athletic endurance decreases. Long-term deficiency in folate intake also leads to easy fatigue and early exhaustion. A survey carried out on a large number of dentists and their wives demonstrated an inverse relationship between average Vitamin C intake and the experience of fatigue. Low Vitamin C-consumption subjects were twice as liable to fatigue symptoms as were the relatively high consumers.

IRON AND TIREDNESS AND FATIGUE

Perhaps the most striking example of fatigue being associated with dietary factors involves iron. In the test described on page 70, those suffering from iron-deficiency anaemia, were clearly more physically affected than those who had sufficient iron in the blood.

MAGNESIUM AND TIREDNESS AND FATIGUE

It is possible that magnesium depletion (a difficult condition to confirm) is associated with a tendency towards chronic tiredness and fatigue. Supplementary magnesium relieved tiredness in 198 out of 200 people, according to a recent survey of magnesium in health and disease.

One really large trial analysis which concentrated on magnesium and potassium in asparate form (see Glossary) showed a pronounced relief in non-specific fatigue of between 75 and 91 per cent in treated patients. The benefit was noticed four to five days after commencing treatment.

GINSENG AND TIREDNESS AND FATIGUE

Ginseng has, as part of its 'adaptogen' function, a reputation for combating fatigue. The product Pharmaton, which contains ginseng as part of its formulation (and also contains

Vitamins A, B group, C, D, E, calcium, bioflavonoids and minerals); would seem an excellent anti-tiredness health food.

COENZYME Q10 AND TIREDNESS AND FATIGUE

Promoted as a recently-discovered 'energy enzyme', this is gaining in repute as an anti-tiredness remedy (see pages 29 – 30).

GOOD BUYS

★ *Gold Standard*
● Iron supplements reinforced by Vitamin C.

Worth Trying
● Ginseng products including Pharmaton (WINDSOR HEALTH-CARE) (see also page 53) ● Coenzyme Q10 ● Magnesium supplements, e.g. Magnesium-OK (WASSEN) ● Vitamin supplements, particularly of B complex.

See also: **Anaemia; Glossary; Immunodepression; Coenzyme Q10; Ginseng; Iron; Magnesium; Potassium; Vitamins B and C.**

VARICOSE VEINS, ULCERS AND HAEMORRHOIDS

BETWEEN 10 and 17 per cent of UK citizens are sufferers from one form of varicose problem or another. Veins can become varicose – swollen and knotted – in several parts of the body. The commonest varicose vein problem is in the legs, in the veins which pump blood back to the heart (against gravity); if the valves in these veins are working less than adequately, blood can collect at certain points and put pressure on and weaken the venous wall.

Veins in the rectum can become varicose as well, and these are known as haemorrhoids, or piles.

In extreme cases of varicose leg veins, varicose ulcers can form on the skin, and these are still one of the major causes of immobility today, especially so far as elderly women are concerned.

Most authorities today believe varicose veins (and piles) are a 'disease' brought about by our ancestors adopting an upright posture, and also pay due deference to genetic factors passing on vein weakness in families. (Indeed, mothers and daughters will often develop varicosities in the same anatomical section of a leg vein at roughly the same ages.)

Signs and Symptoms

Varicose leg veins can produce aching legs, or swollen ankles. They are most common in those who stand a lot (walking *helps* the blood flow in the veins of the legs), and in those who are overweight. Pregnant women can develop them too.

Haemorrhoids are usually the result of undue straining during defaecation, especially when constipated. These can cause pain, bleeding and itching.

A special form of dermatitis – varicose eczema – can appear on the legs, along the line of the varicose vein. The skin becomes dry, shiny and itchy, and may break and develop into an ulcer. This eats into the tissues, and causes pain and bleeding.

Orthodox Medical Management

This is almost entirely a surgical matter – with varicose leg veins being 'stripped'. Injection therapy is usually successful. With haemorrhoids, surgery is occasionally necessary.

Varicose ulcers, once established, are difficult to manage, and dermatologists, general practitioners and surgeons spend much time and effort in the often unrewarding business of trying to persuade them to heal.

Good Health-Food Management

Health foods have been minimally involved in varicose management, and can claim some modest successes. See also Bioflavonoids in the Glossary.

ZINC AND VARICOSE ULCERS

Zinc has proved itself useful not only so far as varicose ulcers are concerned, but in relation to a rather different type of ulcer, the bed (or pressure) sore, a condition common in the bedridden and the paraplegic patient who has to spend most of life in a wheelchair. Professor Derek Bryce-Smith, co-author of *The Zinc Solution* (Century Arrow, 1986), quotes many studies which show that zinc speeds up ulcer healing, whether bed sore or varicose.

The *Lancet* published a double blind study nearly 20 years ago that demonstrated zinc supplements (200mg thrice daily of zinc sulphate) healed varicose ulcers in patients that were zinc-deficient. Other studies have confirmed this but at such high doses toxicity may be a problem. It seems likely that many more of us are zinc-deficient than is suspected, and that health food therapy is under-used in this context (see Zinc).

FIBRE AND VARICOSE PROBLEMS

One particular surgeon (T.L. Cleave) believed that repeatedly striving to pass a constipated stool was the primary cause for leg as well as rectal veins becoming varicose, and advocated a high-fibre diet as a health-food prophylactic. This idea has not gained a large following.

However, fibre does prevent constipation, which may diminish the risks of developing haemorrhoids. Once the problem is established, a fibre-rich diet which softens stools (by retaining water in them) will help relieve pain on defaecation.

GOOD BUYS

- Zinc supplements (e.g. Zinc, 10mg (HEALTHCRAFTS).

Worth Trying
- Fibre products.

See also: **Bed Sores; Bioflavonoids** (Glossary); **Fibre; Zinc.**

Part Three

Appendix
Pharmafax
Addresses
Glossary
References

APPENDIX

A Sensible Dietary Lifestyle

A sensible dietary lifestyle probably involves an element of change, and changing the way you eat – your food lifestyle – needs some effort and a sense of personal commitment.

Approximately one person in three is overweight due to a mis-match of energy (calories) *absorbed* from food and energy *expended* in everyday existence. Obesity is a major risk factor in the development of cardiovascular disease, diabetes, cancer, and high blood pressure. But this mis-match does not just foster obesity. It also tends to foster inadequate mineral and antioxidant intake.

A six-point plan to eat more sensibly is very simple:

1. Increase your daily intake of fruits and vegetables

Ideally, at least one-third of your daily intake should be of raw or very lightly-cooked vegetables or fruit. These contain many nutrients, as well as carbohydrate and fibre (which takes away feelings of hunger).

2. Increase your daily intake of whole-grain foods

Whole-grain cereals, breads and pastas – and pulses as well – are less processed than 'white' equivalents, and therefore contain more nutrients. They are also a healthier source of carbohydrate and fibre.

3. Reduce your daily intake of refined or processed sugars

Many of us eat our weight in sugar and sweetmeats every year – most of it unconsciously, for sugar is a hidden ingredient in masses of commercial foods, such as ham, tinned vegetables, commercial cereals, cakes, biscuits and so on. A high proportion of our unconscious 'sugar' consumption comes from soft drinks, although alcohol also makes a substantial 'sugar' contribution too, comprising 10 per cent of the average social drinking man's and 7.5 per cent of the average woman's calorie intake.

The aim should be to limit sugar calories to 10 per cent of the total daily calorie intake of your diet. Reduction of sugar eating by about 45 per cent should be aimed for, and is not all that difficult to achieve.

4. Reduce overall fat consumption

Fat is Nature's high-density calorie pack. The easiest practical ways to reduce consumption of it are:

- Limit meat portions to 75–100g (3–4oz) meat per day. Choose lean cuts. Cut visible fat off before cooking. Combine with whole-grain pastas, rice, beans etc., to make it go further and look more substantial.

- Do not fry or sauté food; this involves extra fat. Grill, microwave, steam or bake in foil.

- Choose white meats in preference to red. Remove poultry skin.

- Try to eat fish at least twice a week. Fish fats are less saturated than meat fats and have the bonus of essential fatty acid content.

- Avoid luncheon meats, sausages, hot dogs, burgers etc., which contain masses of hidden fat, and fat bacon.

- Limit butter and margarine consumption to two 'pat-size' portions per day. Cook with polyunsatured oils and monounsaturated olive oil, using as little as possible.

- Avoid hidden fat sources such as cakes, biscuits, ice cream, custard, cream, chocolate and pizzas. Look at ready-cooked meals with a healthy suspicion – they often have a high fat content. Limit anything of this nature to, at most, 25g (1oz) per day.

- Drink semi-skimmed milk and eat low-fat cheese. The *fat* content is lower, but the calcium content remains the same.

5. Avoid a too-high intake of sodium
Salt, like sugar, is hidden in many processed foods. Avoid adding at table, using just a little when cooking. Add herbs and other flavourings to bring out taste instead of salt.

6. Work out a sensible nutrient top-up routine
Do this to suit you, or to cater for the symptoms you wish to lose, using the advice this book provides.

PHARMAFAX

The Pharmafax is your guide to the main health food supplements commonly found in the UK today. It does not attempt to give each manufacturer's entire range of products, as this information alone would fill a book.

Inclusion in the Pharmafax is not an endorsement of a product, nor a guarantee of its availability. It should be used in conjunction with Parts One and Two of this book, where you *will* find specific recommendations.

The manufacturers' names appear on the left, and the products' on the right.

Abbreviations Used

caps	capsules	**mg**	milligram
CLO	cod liver oil	**MV**	multivitamin
EPO	evening primrose oil	**NTR**	natural time release
g	gram	**OAD**	one-a-day
HP	high potency	**PR**	prolonged release
HS	high strength	**PRN**	prolonged release
iu	international unit		nutrition
loz.	lozenges	**tabs**	tablets
M	minerals	**TR**	timed release
µg	microgram	**Vit./Vits**	Vitamin(s)

VITAMINS

Vitamin A and Beta-carotene

BLACKMORE'S	Vit. A tabs
BOOTS	Beta carotene
FOOD SUPPLEMENT COMPANY (FSC)	Beta Plus (Natural Beta-carotene + Vits A, C, E, + selenium)
HEALTHCRAFTS	Natural Beta-carotene
	Super Vit. A
HEALTHILIFE	Vit. A caps
	Beta-carotene caps
NATURAL FLOW	Vit. A
	Beta-carotene
QUEST	Beta-carotene
SEVEN SEAS	Natural Beta-carotene caps

Vitamin B

BLACKMORE'S	Vit. B_1
	Vit. B_2
	Vit. B_3
	Vit. B_6
	Vit. B_{12}
BOOTS	Folic Acid
	Vit. B Complex tabs
CANTASSIUM	Folic Acid
	Biotin
	Vit. B_1
	Vit. B_2
	Nicotinamide B_3
	Vit. B_6
	Vit. B_{12}
HEALTHCRAFTS	Compleat Vit. B
	HP Vit. B_6
	PRN Mega B_6
	TR B_6
	Super Brewer's Yeast
	Vit. B_{12}
HEALTHILIFE	Thiamin B_1
	Riboflavin B_2

HOLLAND & BARRETT	Vit. B Complex
	HP Vit. B Complex
	Vit B_6 tabs
	Natural Brewer's Yeast
NATURAL FLOW	Folic Acid
	Vit. B_3 Niacin
	Vit. B_3 Niacinamide
	Biotin/Folic Acid
QUEST	Mega B-50
	Multi B Complex
	Vit. B_6
	Vit. B_{12}
ROCHE	Becosym tabs
	Benerva
	Berocca Effervescent (B group + C + Calcium)
	Sanatogen B_6
	Sanatogen B Complex
SEVEN SEAS	Super B_6 caps
	B Complex with Brewer's Yeast

Vitamin B Plus

AMERICAN NUTRITION (HEALTHCRAFTS)	Strezz B-Vite
BLACKMORE'S	B Complex with Brewer's Yeast
CANTASSIUM	B Complex with Vit. C
	Kalm B Supplement (formerly Stress B Supplement)
HEALTHCRAFTS	PRN Mega-B Complex
	PRN Mega Multi's
	PRN B-Complex with C
	Strezz B-Vite
	TR Vit. B Complex
LAMBERTS	Strezz B-Vite
NATURAL FLOW	Mega B Complex
QUEST	Mega B-50
	Super Mega B + C
VITALIA	Relax B +

Vitamin C

BLACKMORE'S	Vit. C (protein coated)
	Bio C
	Citrus C with Acerola
BOOTS	Vit. C
	Vit. C Chewable
	Effervescent Vit. C
	Vit. C Powder
CANTASSIUM	Vit. C Pure Powder
	Vit. C with Rosehips and Acerola
	Vit. C Chewable
	Vit. C + E
	Rutin
FOOD SUPPLEMENT (FSC) COMPANY	Vit. C with Bioflavonoids
HEALTHCRAFTS	Chewable Vit. C
	HP Vit. C with Bioflavonoids
	Super Vit. C
	Vit. C
	PRN Mega-C
	Vit. C + Zinc
	Vit. C and E Combination
HEALTHILIFE	Chewable Vit. C
	Rutin
	Vit. C with Bioflavinoids
HEALTHWISE	Vit. (with Bioflavonoids)
HOLLAND & BARRETT	HP Vit. C
	Vit. C tabs with Bioflavonoids
	Vit. C Powder
NATURAL FLOW	Super C Complex with Bioflavonoids
	Super C
	Mega C
	Rutin
QUEST	Buffered Vit. C
	Chewable Vit. C
	Vit. C and Bioflavonoids
	Vit. C TR

ROCHE	Redoxon C tabs
	Redoxon Chewable
	Redoxon C Effervescent tabs
	Sanatogen Vit. C tabs
SEVEN SEAS	High Vit. C 'Berries'
	Vit. C-Plus caps

Vitamin A combined with D

QUEST	Vits. A + D
SEVEN SEAS	Natural Vits. A + D caps

Vitamin E

BLACKMORE'S	Vit. E range (tabs and caps)
BOOTS	Chewable Vit. E
	Natural Vit. E
CANTASSIUM	Vit. E (natural)
HEALTHCRAFTS	Vit. E
	Super Vit. E
	Water-Soluble Vit. E
	HP Vit. E
	Mega Vit. E
HEALTHILIFE	Vit. E caps
HOLLAND & BARRETT	Vit. E
LANES	Fort-E-Vite
NATURAL FLOW	Vit. E
QUEST	Vit. E Natural Ratio Mixed Tocopherols
	Vit. E 100% Δ Alpha Tocopherol
ROCHE	Ephynal tabs
	Sanatogen Vit. E caps
SEVEN SEAS	Super Vit. E caps
	Natural Vit. E in Wheatgerm Oil caps

Multivitamins

BLACKMORE'S	Bio Ace
BOOTS	MV
	Effervescent MV
	MV + Iron
	MV, M + Ginseng
CANTASSIUM	Vitamins and Minerals with EPO
HEALTHCRAFTS	Chewable MV
	MV + Iron
	MV + Iron + Calcium
	Vits. A,C,D
	PRN Mega Multi's
HOLLAND & BARRETT	MV + M tabs
	MV + Iron tabs
	MV + Vit. C tabs
	HP MV tabs
	HP MV + M (for vegetarians)
QUEST	Improved OAD MV + Chelated M
	Super OAD TR MV + Chelated M
ROCHE	Sanatogen MV + Calcium
	Sanatogen MV + EPO caps
	Sanatogen MV + M
	Santogen MV + Iron
SEVEN SEAS	Minadex Children's Vit. A, C + D tabs
	Minadex MV Syrup
	MV from Natural Sources OAD
	MV from Natural Sources + Iron OAD
	MV + M + Ginseng caps
	MV + M caps
	MV with EPO
VITALIFE	Multiplus V + M + Ginseng
WASSEN	Genesis (MV, M, Iron)

MINERALS AND MICRONUTRIENTS

Calcium

BIO HEALTH	Extra Calcium
BLACKMORES	Chewable Calcium
	Bio Calcium
BOOTS	Chewable Calcium
	Calcium + Vit. D caps or chewable
CANTASSIUM	Dolomite (with magnesium)
	Calcimega
CEDAR HEALTH	Porosis D
ENGLISH GRAINS HEALTHCARE	Calcia
FOOD SUPPLEMENT COMPANY (FSC)	Calcium Magnesium and Zinc
	Super Dolomite
HEALTHCRAFTS	Aminochel Calcium
	Chewable Calcium
	Dolomite (with magnesium)
	PRN Calcium Pantothenate
	Super Calcium Plus
LIFEPLAN	Magnezie (with magnesium + Vits + Mins) OAD
	Caltabs
	Dolomite (with Magnesium)
NATURAL FLOW	Calcium-Magnesium
	Dolomite with Vits. A + D
QUEST	Balanced Ratio Cal-Mag (+ Vit. D)
SEVEN SEAS	Calcium 'Berries' with Vit. D
VITABIOTICS	Osteocare

Iron

ABBOTT	Ferrograd
ASTA MEDICA	Ferrocontin Continus
BLACKMORE'S	Iron Compound
BOOTS	Iron + Vit. C tabs
	Vitamins + Iron Syrup
FOOD SUPPLEMENT COMPANY (FSC)	Blackstrap Molasses Iron (+ Vit. C)
HEALTHCRAFTS	Aminochel Iron
	Iron Plus
	MV and Iron
	MV with Iron + Calcium
LANES	Maxivit MV + M tabs
QUEST	Multiminerals
	Synergistic Iron
SANATOGEN	MV plus Iron
SEVEN SEAS	Minadex MV Syrup
	Minadex Children's Vit. A, C + D tabs
	Minadex Orange Flavour Tonic
	Iron 'Berries' with Vit. C
VITABIOTICS	Ferus B_{12}
	Multiron
	Feroglobin (Iron, Minerals + Vit. B)
WASSEN	Genesis (MV + Iron)

Magnesium

HEALTHCRAFTS	Aminochel Magnesium
LIFEPLAN	Magnezie (Magnesium, Calcium, Zinc + Vits + Mins) OAD
QUEST	Synergistic Magnesium
SEVEN SEAS	Magnesium 'Berries'
WASSEN	Magnesium-OK

Potassium

CANTASSIUM	Potassium B_{13}
NATURAL FLOW	Potassium
NATURE'S OWN	Potassium

Selenium

BOOTS	Selenium + Vit. E
CANTASSIUM	Selenium Supplement
	Yeast-free Selenium
HOLLAND & BARRETT	Selenium
LIFEPLAN	Selenium Bonus (+ Vits + Mins)
NATURAL FLOW	Selenium
	Super Selenium Compound
QUEST	Synergistic Selenium
SEVEN SEAS	Selenium with Vit. E in CLO
WASSEN	Selenium-ACE

Zinc

BLACKMORES	Bio Zinc
BOOTS	Chewable zinc + Vit. C
	Zinc caps
CANTASSIUM	Zinc with M
	Zinc + B_6
	Zinc B13
	Zinc + B_6 drops
FOOD SUPPLEMENT	Zinc (elemental 4mg)
COMPANY (FSC)	Zinc Picolinate
	Zinc loz. + Vit. C + Peppermint
	Aminochel Zinc
HEALTHCRAFTS	Vit. C + Zinc
	Zinc
	HP Aminochel Zinc

HEALTHILIFE	Zinc
	Mega Zinc loz.
HEALTHRITE	Zinc Gluconate
HOLLAND & BARRETT	Chelated Zinc
NATURAL FLOW	Zinc
	Chewable Zinc
QUEST	Synergistic Zinc
SEVEN SEAS	Zinc 'Berries' with Vit. C
THAMES	Solvazinc
VITALIA	Zincold 23 (+ Vit. C)

PLANT OILS

Evening Primrose Oil (EPO)

BOOTS	EPO
	EPO chewable
	EPO with Fish Oil
	EPO + Royal Jelly
BRITANNIA HEALTH	Oil of Evening Primrose
	Efavite
	Efamol
	Efamol Oil
	Efamol Marine (marine oil with EPO + Vit. E)
	Efamol Plus (EPO, safflower and linseed oils, + Vit. E)
CANTASSIUM	Primrose AC + E
	Super GLA
EVENING PRIMROSE OIL COMPANY (EPOC)	EPO caps
	EPOC Marine (pure EPO + Marine fish oil with Vit. E)
	EPOC Liquid (pure EPO with Vit. E)

HEALTHCRAFTS	Oil of Evening Primrose caps
	EPO Forte
HEALTHILIFE	EPO
HOLLAND & BARRETT	EPO caps
LIFEPLAN	Galanol GLX EPO
	Galanol Gold (EPO enriched with GLA)
NATURAL FLOW	EPO
QUEST	Gammaoil Premium
ROCHE	Sanatogen EPO
SEVEN SEAS	EPO 'Berries' + Vit. E
	HS EPO with Borage Oil
	Super EPO with GLA
	Pure CLO with EPO
	Almond Oil with Borage Oil + Vits A, D and E
VITALIA	EPO + Salmon Oil

Other Plant Oils

G & G	Cold-Pressed Linseed Oil caps
HEALTHILIFE	Sunflower Seed Oil caps
	Safflower Seed Oil caps
LANES	Glanolin (blackcurrant seed oil)
LIFEPLAN	Super Galanol (oil of borage)
	Super Galanol (starflower oil)
ROCHE	Starflower Oil

MARINE OILS

Cod Liver Oil

BLACKMORE'S	CLO caps
BOOTS	CLO caps
	OAD CLO
CANTASSIUM	CLO caps
	OAD CLO caps

HEALTHCRAFTS	CLO caps
	Compleat CLO
	Arterol
HEALTHILIFE	Pure CLO (caps and liquid)
	HS CLO caps
HOLLAND & BARRETT	Cod Liver Oil OAD caps
NATURAL FLOW	EPA
QUEST	Pure CLO HS
ROCHE	Sanatogen CLO
	Sanatogen CLO caps
	Sanatogen CLO + MV caps
SEVEN SEAS	Pure CLO
	Pure CLO caps
	Pure CLO HS OAD
	Pure CLO with EPO
	Orange Syrup + CLO
	Lemon Flavour Pure CLO Spoonful

Other Marine Oils

BOOTS	Halibut Liver Oil caps
CANTASSIUM	Mega Fish Oil (with shark and salmon liver oils)
HEALTHCRAFTS	Super Seatone
	Super Halibut Liver Oil
HEALTHILIFE	Pure Halibut Liver Oil
LANES	Lanepa (concentrated Omega 3 fish oil), caps and liquid
NOVEX	MAXEPA (Omega 3 marine triglycerides)
QUEST	Gamma EPA (fish oil concentrate)
	Gamma Marine (EPO, borage and fish oils)
ROCHE	Sanatogen Pure Fish Oils caps

SEVEN SEAS	Pulse Pure Fish Oils caps
	Pure Fish Oils and Kelp caps
VITABIOTICS	Omega H3
VITALIA	Epopa (Omega 6, Omega 3, safflower, salmon, EPO, borage, Vit. E, niacin)
WASSEN	Omega-3 Fish Oil

OTHER PRODUCTS

Garlic

BLACKMORE'S	Garlix
	Garlic Oil
	Odourless Garlic
BOOTS	Garlic Oil
	Odourless OAD Garlic Oil
CANTASSIUM	Garlic Oil caps
	Garlimega
HEALTHCRAFTS	Odourless Garlic
	OAD Garlic Pearles
	Odourless Garlic Pearles
HEALTHILIFE	OAD Odourless Mega Garlic Pearls
	OAD Odourless Garlic Pearls
	Odourless Garlic Pearls
HÖFELS	Garlic and Parsley OAD tabs
	Garlic Pearles OAD
	Odourless Neo Garlic Pearles OAD
	Cardiomax Garlic Pearles OAD
HOLLAND & BARRETT	OAD Garlic Perles
	Garlic Perles Odourless
LANES	Lusty's Garlic Perles

LICHTWER PHARMA	Kwai Highly Concentrated Garlic tabs
QUEST	Kyolic range
	Kyolic Liquid
ROCHE	Sanatogen OAD Garlic Perles
SEVEN SEAS	Garlic Oil Perles
	Odourless Garlic Oil Perles
VITALIA	Garlic High Potency
	Garlic Odourless
WASSEN	OAD (delayed diffusion) Garlic tabs

Ginseng

BLACKMORE'S	Ginseng tabs
BOOTS	Korean Ginseng
CANTASSIUM	Red Panax Ginseng
	Red Ginseng
ENGLISH GRAINS HEALTHCARE	Red Kooga (caps, tabs, elixir)
HEALTHCRAFTS	HP Korean Ginseng
	HP Siberian Ginseng
	Korean-Siberian Ginseng Combination
	GEB_6 (Siberian Ginseng + Vits. E + B_6)
	Mega Korean Ginseng
HOLLAND & BARRETT	Korean Ginseng caps
	HP Ginseng
POWER HEALTH	Power Ginseng GX 2500
ROCHE	Sanatogen Korean Ginseng
SEVEN SEAS	Korean Ginseng caps
WINDSOR HEALTHCARE	Pharmaton caps

Pollen, Propolis and Royal Jelly

BOOTS	Royal Jelly
BRITANNIA HEALTH	Prostabrit (Cernilton)
CANTASSIUM	Propolis loz.

FOOD SUPPLEMENT COMPANY (FSC)	HP Propolis Propolis Tincture
HEALTHCRAFTS	Super Royal Jelly HP Royal Jelly
HOLLAND & BARRETT	Royal Jelly
SANATOGEN	Royal Jelly
SEVEN SEAS	Royal Jelly 'Berries' Royal Jelly with Natural Propolis + Honey
VITALIA	Royal Jelly
WASSEN	Pollen-B

High-fibre Products

ARCOCAPS	Fibre Time 400 Phytofibre
BLACKMORE'S	Apple Fibre Chewable Complex
BOOTS	Multi Fibre tabs
FINK	Linusit Gold
GRANNY ANN	High Fibre Biscuits
JORDANS	Natural Country Bran Oat Bran
NUTRICIA DIETARY PRODUCTS	GF Dietary Beta-Fibre Rite-Diet High Fibre Bread

Women's Specialities

BRITANNIA HEALTH	Efamol Pre-Menstrual Pack
CANTASSIUM	Acidophilus tabs
GOLDSHIELD PHARMACEUTICALS	Pregnavite Forte F
HEALTHCRAFTS	PRN Mega Multi's
LADYCARE (HEALTHCRAFTS)	Monthly Menopause Post Menopause

LAMBERTS	Acidophilus Extra
NATURE'S OWN	Acidophilus
NATURAL FLOW	Acidophilus
PARKWOOD HEALTH (HEALTHCRAFTS)	Gynovite Plus
QUEST	Non-Dairy Acidophilus Plus
VITABIOTICS	Menopace
	Ladytone
	Osteocare
WASSEN	Confiance
	Magnesium-OK

Unclassified Products

CANTASSIUM	Kelp Plus 3
COLGATE-PALMOLIVE	Fluorigard
DENTAL HEALTH	Fluor-a-Day
FSC	Sea Kelp and Potassium
HEALTHCRAFTS	Feverfew tabs
	Kelp Plus
	Night Time
HEALTHILIFE	Sea Kelp
	Co-Q-10
HEALTHWISE	Feverfew
HOLLAND & BARRETT	Feverfew tabs
	Kelp with Added Calcium
	LAB Laboprin (lycine + aspirin sachets)
	Goodnite tabs
LANES	Lanes Co-Q-10
LIFEPLAN	Feverfew caps
NATURE'S OWN	Brewers' Yeast
NATURAL FLOW	Coenzyme Q10

NOVEX	Mintec (peppermint oil)
QUEST	Feverfew (leaves)
	Coenzyme Q10
TILLOTTS	Colperin (peppermint oil)
VITALIA	Sea Kelp
WASSEN	Sitosteroil-B (beta sitosteroil, Vit. A, niacin, Vits. B,C,E, selenium, chromium)
	Coenzyme Q10 (+ Vit. E)

ADDRESSES

Most manufacturers are happy to answer queries about their products. Some offer a mail order service.

Abbott Laboratories Ltd, Abbot House, Norden Rd, Maidenhead, Berks SL6 4XE   Tel: 0628 773355

ASTA Medica Ltd, 168 Cowley Road, Cambridge, Cambs. CB4 4DL   Tel: 0223 423434

Bio-Health Ltd, Culpeper Close, Medway City Estate, Rochester, Kent ME2 4HU   Tel: 0634 290115

Blackmore's Laboratories Ltd, Unit 7, Poyle, Colnbrook, Bucks SL3 0PD   Tel: 0753 683815

Boots Pharmaceuticals UK, 9 Castle Quay, Castle Boulevard, Nottingham, Notts. NG7 IFW   Tel: 0602 498335

Britannia Health Products Ltd, Forum Holdings, Forum House, 41–51 Brighton Road, Redhill, Surrey RH1 6YS   Tel: 0737 773741

Cantassium, Larkhill Laboratories, 225 Putney Bridge Road, London SW15 2PY   Tel: 081 874 1130

Cedar Health Ltd, Pepper Road, Hazel Grove, Stockport, Cheshire SK7 5BW   Tel: 061 483 1235

Colgate-Palmolive Ltd, Guildford Business Park, Middleton Road, Guildford, Surrey GU2 5LZ   Tel: 0483 302222

Dental Health Products Ltd, Torbet Laboratories, Broughton House, 33 Earl Street, Maidstone, Kent ME14 1PF   Tel: 0622 762269

English Grains Holdings Ltd, Swains Park Industrial Estate, Park Road, Overseal, Swadlincote, Derbyshire DE12 6JT   Tel: 0283 221616

Evening Primrose Oil Company, c/o Norgine Ltd, 116–120 London Road, Headington, Oxford OX3 9BA   Tel: 0865 750717

Food Supplement Company (FSC), c/o Health & Diet Company, Ltd, Europa Park, Stoneclough Road, Radcliffe, Manchester M26 1GG   Tel: 0204 707420

G & G Foods Supplies Ltd, 175 London Road, East Grinstead, West Sussex RH19 1YY   Tel: 0342 312811

Goldshield Pharmaceuticals Ltd, Bensham House, 324 Bensham Lane, Thornton Heath, Surrey CR7 7EQ   Tel: 081 684 3664

Healthcrafts, Ferroson Healthcare Ltd, Beaver House, York Close, Byfleet, Surrey KT14 7HN   Tel: 0932 336366

Healthilife Ltd, Charlestown House, Baildon, Shipley, West Yorkshire BD17 7JS   Tel: 0274 595021

Healthrite, Abbots Close, Oyster Lane, Byfleet, Surrey, KT14 7JP Tel. 0932 354211

Healthwise, York House, York St, Bradford, W Yorks. BD8 0HR Tel 0274 488511

Holland & Barrett, Unit 1, Dodwells Road, Dodwells Bridge Industrial Estate, Hinckley, Leics. LE10 3B2   Tel: 0455 251900

Jordan, W. (Cereals) Ltd, Holme Mills, Biggleswade, Beds. SG18 9JX   Tel: 0767 318222

LAB (Laboratories for Applied Biology Ltd), 91 Amhurst Park, London N16 5DR   Tel: 081 800 2252

Lamberts Healthcare Ltd, 1 Lamberts Road, Tunbridge Wells, Kent TN2 3EQ   Tel: 0892 546488

Lane, G.R., Health Products Ltd, Sisson Road, Gloucester GL1 3QB   Tel: 0452 524012

Lichtwer Pharma UK, Dominions House, Eton Place, 64 High Street, Burnham, Bucks. SL1 7JT   Tel: 0628 605275

Lifeplan Products Ltd, Elizabethan Way, Lutterworth, Leics. LE17 4ND   Tel: 0455 556281

Natural Flow, Larkhall Laboratories, 225 Putney Bridge Road, London SW15 2PY   Tel: 081 874 1130

Nature's Own, 203 West Malvern Road, West Malvern, Worcs. WR14 4BB   Tel: 0684 982555

Novex Pharma, Division of Innovex Ltd, Innovex House, 309 Reading Road, Henley-on-Thames, Oxon. RG9 1EL   Tel: 0491 578171

Nutricia Dietary Products Ltd, 494–496 Honeypot Lane, Stanmore, Middlesex HA7 1JR   Tel: 081 951 5155

Potters, Leyland Mill Lane, Wigan, Lancs. WN1 2SB   Tel: 0942 34761

Power Health Products Ltd, 10 Central Avenue, Airfield Estate, Pocklington, North Yorks YO4 2NR   Tel: 0759 302595

Quest Vitamins Ltd, Unit 1, Premier Trading Estate, Dartmouth Middleway, Birmingham B7 4AT   Tel: 021 359 0056

Roche Products Ltd, PO Box 8, Broadwater Road, Welwyn Garden City, Herts. AL7 3AY   Tel: 0707 366000

Scotia Pharmaceuticals Ltd, Woodbridge Meadows, Guildford, Surrey GU1 1BA   Tel: 0483 574949

Seven Seas Ltd, Marfleet, Kingston-upon-Hull, Humberside HU9 5NJ   Tel: 0482 75234

Thames Laboratories Ltd, Abbey House, Wrexham Industrial Estate, Wrexham, Clwyd LL13 9PW   Tel: 0978 661351

Tillotts Laboratories, c/o The Pharmacia, Davy Avenue, Knowl Hill, Milton Keynes MK5 8PH   Tel: 0908 661101

Vitabiotics Ltd, Vitabiotics House, 3 Bashley Road, London NW10 6SU   Tel: 081 963 0999

Vitalia Ltd, Paradise, Hemel Hempstead, Herts. HP2 4TF   Tel: 0442 231155

Wassen International Ltd, 14 The Mole Business Park, Leatherhead, Surrey KT22 7BA   Tel: 0372 379828

Windsor Healthcare Ltd, Ellesfield Avenue, Bracknell, Berks RG12 8YS   Tel: 0344 484448

GLOSSARY

AMINO ACIDS

These are complex organic molecules from which our body builds even more complex proteins that make up our muscles and bodies generally. They are the small 'building blocks' of protein. Science traditionally divides amino acids into essential and non-essential: the former have to be eaten to become part of us, while the latter can be synthesised within the body.

Interest from the health-food point of view centres on *Lysine*, which is used for recurrent cold sores and herpes infections (see page 238), and *Taurine*, the possible uses for which include dementia prophylaxis. *Tyrasine* is used experimentally in Parkinson's Disease; *Tryptophan* was at one time found to be useful in the treatment of depression, but is now under a cloud, probably because one Japanese pharmaceutical source was contaminated and produced devastating side effects. *Arginine* is thought to improve fertility in men, and *L-Histidine* was hailed as an anti-rheumatic, but not supported by an experimental double blind study.

It is possible that amino acids will become more popular in terms of health-food interest as time passes, provided good experimental evidence evolves relative to their therapeutic action.

ANTIOXIDANTS AND FREE RADICALS

Antioxidants are a group of unrelated chemical substances present in many foods, which play an important part in protecting various tissues in the body from substances called free radicals. The micronutrient selenium and the Vitamins A (beta-carotene), C and E are antioxidants. To understand their importance, we have to enter the world of atomic and molecular chemistry.

We need to breathe oxygen to keep us alive. We use it

321

internally to produce the energy we need to keep our bodies going. Mostly we use oxygen as the main currency of biological energy and we convert it into carbon dioxide and water. But not *all* the oxygen in the air we breathe finishes up as this. A normal oxygen atom has four pairs of electrons. A variety of biological processes can rob the oxygen atom of an electron. It is now a *free radical* whose chemical ambition is to replace the lost electron by raiding other molecules. This raid can erode the walls of cells, changing their character and opening the door to various disease processes. Antioxidants 'tame' these free radicals.

However, once free radicals are liberated they can do considerable damage to tissues and nutrients before the body limits their power by the mobilisation of antioxidants. In a state of biological harmony antioxidants in the diet make sure that free radicals produced in excess of demand are effectively mopped up before they can damage our tissues. Usually the body does this quickly and efficiently, providing it has an adequate and mobile bank of antioxidants at its disposal.

Ageing and many of the so-called degenerative diseases (artery problems, cancer, arthritis and rheumatism, for instance) can be caused and exacerbated by free-radical damage. Dietary supplementation with antioxidants is important, and health foods can help prevent this damage.

ASPARTATE

A derivative of aspartic acid which is a nonessential amino acid occuring naturally in sugar cane and sugar beat.

ATOPIC
Allergic.

BETA-BLOCKERS

These reduce response of the heart to stress and exercise. They are used to treat angina to lower blood pressure and to correct abnormal rhythms.

BETA-CAROTENE

Beta-carotene is a Vitamin A-type substance that occurs in vegetables. Vitamin A 'proper' is only found in animal products. The body can produce Vitamin A from beta-carotene. Beta-carotene is soluble in water and so does not get stored in the body as does Vitamin A. Excess Vitamin A can be toxic, whereas excess beta-carotene seldom causes problems other than making the skin look yellow.

BIOFLAVONOIDS

The bioflavonoids are something of a 'mixed bag' of nutrients which were discovered in Hungarian red peppers in the 1930s and were, for a time, called Vitamin P. For several years they were believed to be capable of acting as a sort of super Vitamin C, and in animal experiments they did seem to clear up Vitamin C deficiency diseases more effectively than Vitamin C.

The only bioflavonoid that appears much in health foods today is *rutin*. Most fruits are rich in bioflavonoids – citrin is contained in citrus fruit – but boiling and storage cause considerable losses. Whether or not there are signs and symptoms of, and therefore diseases due to, bioflavonoid deficiency seems to be a moot point. At one time there was enthusiasm for bioflavonoids as a cure for the common cold but a properly controlled double blind trial involving 2000 people was negative. Another enthusiasm for the bioflavonoids held sway for some time in the management of purpura (spontaneous bleeding in the skin), but this was blunted when results were not confirmed.

It might be convenient to forget about bioflavonoids in the health-food marketplace were it not for three interesting trials.

1. Ménière's disease is an unpleasant condition characterised by deafness, vertigo and tinnitus (ringing in the ears). Conventional medical treatment is often far from helpful. In one trial, 600mg of citrus bioflavonoids daily improved hearing and reduced vertigo. Diarrhoea was experienced as a side effect.

2. Varicose veins and their complications often lead to profound disability and morbidity (see page 294). Double blind

studies (the sort that impress doctors!) have demonstrated beneficial effects of bioflavonoids in the treatment of varicose veins and related conditions.

3. Dr Thomas Stuttaford, *The Times'* trusted medical columnist, recently (28.10.93) drew readers' attention to research in *The Lancet* that suggested that flavonoids in tea, red wine and apples are cardio protective and that research is preceeding to investigate claims that green tea protects against malignant disease.

BLIND TRIAL

A medical trial in which patients do not know if they are taking the substance under trial or an inert substance (see Placebo, below). See also Double Blind Trial (below).

BIO-AVAILABILITY

A term used to explain the concept of a food being able to contribute towards the biologic process. Some foods can pass through the gut virtually unchanged. These have a low bio-availability.

CHELATION

Chelation produces very stable 'ring-structured' compounds of considerable pharmalogical value.

CHELATING AGENTS

These are capable of forming a chemical complexity with (usually) a metallic substance present in the body in unwanted concentrations so that it can slowly but effectively be excreted.

CHOLESTEROL

A complex alcoholic substance involved in many body functions, which is present in the blood normally up to 200mg per 100cc of blood.

CROSS LINKING

The progressive formation of chemical bonds as bridges between large molecules, particularly proteins. Cross linkings results in a loss of tissue flexibility. It is seen in ageing skin and in ageing inorganic substances, e.g. old windscreen wipers, plastics, hot water bottles. Free radicals, chemicals and sunlight can promote cross linking in animal tissues.

Δ-ALPHA TOCOPHEROL

A natural form of Vitamin E.

DOUBLE BLIND TRIAL

A medical trial in which neither patients nor trial organiser know whether the patient is taking a test substance or placebo until the trial code is 'broken' and evaluation commences.

DYSPLASIA

Abnormal tissue formation.

ENTERIC-COATED PREPARATIONS

Manufactured so that they pass through the stomach intact, to be liberated in the intestine.

ESSENTIAL FATTY ACIDS (EFAs)

Just after the First World War, one of the discoveries in the exciting new world of nutritional science was that all fats were chemically rather similar – consisting of varying combinations of glycerol (glycerine) and substances called fatty acids. (Some of these fatty acids got their names from the fat on your plate: a pat of butter contains butyric acid; a spoonful of olive oil gets its flavour and consistency from oleic acid.)

Much later, food scientists stumbled upon another new nutritional concept – the idea of *essentiality* applied to certain rather special fatty acids. These *essential* fatty acids (or EFAs) are polyunsaturated fats which are necessary in the body – for food metabolism – but which, like many vitamins and minerals, cannot be manufactured in the body and have to be provided in the diet. If they are lacking in the diet, signs of deficiency occur.

The primary function of EFAs is to keep the prostaglandin action functional. The prostaglandins are hormone-like messengers, vital to the health of the body, which are synthesised from EFAs. They are being made in the body all the time, so we need a constant supply of essential fatty acids, as the body does not store the latter.

Gradually it was found that there are several types of these essential fatty acids. Marine oils, and particularly cod liver oil, are rich in EFAs. Another interesting group is the plant oil-derived EFAs, which include linoleic acid, found in large amounts in many vegetable seed oils, and linolenic acid, found in linseed and many plant leaves (the name comes from linseed).

TWO VERY IMPORTANT VEGETABLE EFAs

Linoleic
Found in large amounts in certain vegetable seeds: safflower 77 per cent; sunflower 65 per cent; soy bean 51 per cent; olive oil 7 per cent. It is the most common polyunsaturated fatty acid in food.

Linolenic
The predominant EFA found in leaf vegetables. Found also in linseed oil (57 per cent) from which it got its name. Is converted in the body to the fish oil type of EFA. One particularly important type of linolenic acid is GLA (gamma linolenic acid).

As knowledge gradually accumulated, it became obvious that among the essential EFAs there lurked something of a nutritional superstar. It was slightly different in its organic chemical configuration from 'ordinary' linolenic acid, and it was subsequently called *gamma* linolenic acid (or GLA for short). GLA was subsequently shown to be ten times more biologically effective than 'ordinary' linolenic acid. Certain plant seed oils, especially evening primrose oil, are the richest source.

The body manufactures its vital GLA by means of a special enzyme called delta-6-desaturase, and it is worthwhile mentioning this because it is at this *enzyme* level in our tissues that various blocking factors can inhibit our GLA production taking place. Among the most common agents which can block GLA products in the body are:

- A diet too rich in saturated animal fat
- Too much alcohol as part of everyday living
- Poorly-controlled diabetes
- Excessive and pointless stress
- The ageing process
- Viral infections (colds, influenza, certain pneumonias).

FREE RADICALS see ANTIOXIDANTS

GAMMA LINOLENIC ACID (GLA)

Formed from linolenic acid. Substantial amounts are found particularly in evening primrose oil. **See also** Essential Fatty Acids.

HAEMOGLOBIN

The respiratory pigments of the red blood corpuscles.

INDICATED

Recommended, judged to be a correct course of action.

MICRONUTRIENTS

These are sometimes called trace elements, or trace minerals, and are so called because only minute quantities are necessary to the body to maintain health. But some of these tiny amounts are absolutely vital. Thousands of children used to die in China each year from heart failure because their diet lacked the micronutrient selenium. When the diet was supplemented with selenium, the disease became a rarity.

Micronutrients are usually measured in micrograms (μg). The smallness of this quantity is difficult to appreciate, but the following may help. Take an ounce (28g) of flour, and divide it into 28 equal portions – each will weigh 1 gram (g). Divide one of these heaps into a thousand equal heaps, and each speck will weigh a milligram (mg). Now divide one milligram speck into a thousand pieces – each will weigh a microgram (µg).

The nutritionally important micronutrients are cobalt, copper, fluoride and selenium (those which have a place in this health-food guide), as well as chromium, manganese and molybdenum.

MINERALS

Derived from the word *mine*, the term covers any inorganic substance formed in nature. But as far as nutrition is concerned these are crystalline chemical elements and compounds required in macro quantities in the diet (several hundreds or indeed thousands of milligrams). Those that are covered nutritionally are calcium, iodine, iron, magnesium, potassium and zinc, but other minerals include phosphorus, chlorine, silicon and sodium.

Although only a tiny proportion of the body weight is actually mineral matter, minerals (and trace minerals, see Micronutrients) are vital for both mental and physical well-being. They are important in the formation and maintenance of many tissues and cells and, like the vitamins, play a part in the chemical interreactions involved in many body processes, such as digestion and respiration.

MITOGEN

Substance that stimulates cell division.

MONOUNSATURATED OILS

Fats with only one degree of saturation e.g. oleic acid which is contained in olive oil in large amounts.

PHYTATE

A salt of phytic acid, a substance which prevents absorption of calcium from the gut. Found in wholemeal flour but partially destroyed if yeast is used in preparation of bread.

PLACEBO

Latin for 'I will please'. There are several ways in which the word is used, e.g. a placebo in a blind trial (see entry above) is an inert substance that physically resembles the substance under trial. A doctor may prescribe a placebo to humour the patient as part and parcel of evey day treatment. Many medical treatments succeed because of the placebo response.

POLYSACCHARIDES

Literally 'many sugars'. Chemists use this term to define a group of carbohydrates that contain more than three simple carbohydrates combined.

POLYUNSATURATED OILS

A concept elaborated to describe the organic chemistry of oils (and fats). Oils and fats are compounds of fatty acids. These are composed of chains of carbon atoms, each of which is linked to hydrogen atoms. When every carbon atom in a fat is linked to a hydrogen atom in all possible positions, this fat is 'saturated' (with hydrogen). In polyunsaturated fats bonding between carbon atoms occurs and this prevents the fat being saturated (with hydrogen). If there is more than one instance of a carbon-to-carbon bond in a fat it is called a polyunsaturated fat. **See also** Monounsaturated Oils.

PRECURSOR SUBSTANCES

When an organism is building up complex organic substances it often does so by using less complex substances as 'building bricks'. These are sometimes referred to as precursor substances. Beta-carotene is a precursor to Vitamin A.

PROGESTERONE

A naturally occuring female sex hormone, responsible, among other things, for the secretory changes in the lining of the uterus in the last two weeks of the menstrual cycle. It is also necessary for maintaining pregnancy.

PROGESTOGEN

Any of a group of steroid hormones that mimic the action of the female sex hormone progesterone. Progestogens are used in oral contraceptive preparations.

PROSPECTIVE STUDY

The researcher alters something and observes what happens (as opposed to a retrospective study in which a change is observed and related to possible alterations).

PROSTAGLANDINS

The prostaglandins are highly biologically active substances with many functions. They play a vital part in the regulation and control of all cell growth and regeneration, as well as the regulation of our immune system and the control of inflammation. They also have an important role to play in the maintaining of the health of the skin and the welfare of the cardiovascular system.

Prostaglandins were originally extracted from the prostate gland, and they were named after that mysterious male gland whose main practical function seems to be to direct the ejaculate at the moment of orgasm in men. However, it soon became obvious that there were many more prostaglandins lurking in different body tissues, and in both sexes. The name may have been wrong, but the prostaglandins are vital to our well-being.

In an attempt to explain just *how* prostaglandins keep us healthy, they have been likened to hormones. Hormones are chemical substances that various glands (the thyroid, ovaries, testes, etc.) in our bodies release into the bloodstream to speed up our metabolism, control growth, modify sexual function, and so on. Prostaglandins do this self-same sort of thing, but in a rather different way, by working *locally* in the tissues. If hormones are the 'flying squad' or biological runners, combating emergency situations, then prostaglandins are the 'policemen on the beat', looking after us and quietly keeping us in order on a more local, tissue-specific basis.

Prostaglandins are manufactured quite locally too, from fatty acids in our food. For one of the prostaglandins' functions is intimately related to the body's use of the common basic foodstuff we think of simply as fat. Our body takes in fat in various chemical forms, and digests it into fatty acids that it subsequently uses in several very distinct and differing ways. It can either 'burn' fat internally to produce energy, store it against time of famine as body fat, or convert some of it into prostaglandins. But it all depends to some extent on the type (or formula) of fat (chemically) that we eat as to exactly what the body *can* do to it in the way of fat utilisation.

The body needs rather special types of food fat – the *essential* fatty acids (EFAs) – before it can make *all* the prostaglandins it needs *all* the time. Something of a breakthrough occurred when it was discovered that EFAs, particularly the linolenic class and GLA (see Essential Fatty Acids), and the Marine Oils were basic foods that can make a very substantial contribution to our health as far as prostaglandin status is concerned. Evening primrose oil and cod liver oil are particularly valuable.

It seems unlikely that prostaglandins are stored to any extent in the tissues that need them, and this implies that our body needs a constant supply of EFAs to generate prostaglandins on demand. This suggests that a regular intake of certain fatty acids may be involved in the prevention, and perhaps the treatment, of various disease states.

PROVITAMIN

Something that the body can convert into a vitamin, e.g. beta-carotene into Vitamin A.

QUINONES

Complex ring-structured organic compounds composed of hydrogen, oxygen and carbon atoms. The best known quinone is Coenzyme Q (CoQ10).

RETINOL

The chemical name for Vitamin A.

SUCCINATE

A salt of succinic acid.

TOCOPHEROL

The chemical name for Vitamin E. It comes in various forms and has been given Greek letters to identify these. δλ alpha tocopherol acetate is the most active of these and vitamin E activity is conventionally stated as such.

TRACE ELEMENTS See MICRONUTRIENTS

VASODILATORS

Drugs that dilate (expand) blood vessels.

VITAMINS

There is no way that we could live a healthy, active and productive life on a diet of pure chemical protein, fat and carbohydrate even if we supplemented it with the necessary minerals and micronutrients. To keep healthy we need to eat plant or animal *tissues* as well, because in those tissues lurk the substances that we know as vitamins. These cannot be manufactured by the body, so have to be supplied by food. We need very small quantities of these each day – in most cases less than 5mg, the weight of a few grains of granulated sugar (although in the case of Vitamin C we need much more, at least 40 – 60mg).

Vitamins are so called because the scientists who discovered them believed they were chemicals called *amines*, and so they coined the word 'vitamin' from the concept of *vital amines*, which became our vitamins. Now we know that vitamins are not amines at all, but the name has stuck!

It is suggested by some that in affluent societies we can forget about vitamins, but this is not true, particularly so far as folate, thiamin and Vitamins C and D are concerned. Various groups of people are particularly vulnerable to vitamin lack. For example, children, the elderly, the institutionalised and drug abusers are at risk, but not so much as those who live socially deprived lives close to the economic breadline, or those who opt for bizarre diets. Finally there is a very difficult group to evaluate – the poor absorbers.

Most nutritionalists recommend food rather than supplements to make sure that vitamin deficiences do not occur. This is a laudable enough diktat provided that we constantly remember how easily foods are depleted of their vitamins. This cannot be stressed too much in this good health-food guide.

REFERENCES

Do you want to know more? Here are the main references used in preparing this book.

INTRODUCTION

Anderson, D., *A Diet of Reason*, Social Affairs Unit, 1986.

Angel, A. and Roncarl, D., 'Medical complications of obesity', *Canadian Medical Association Journal*, 1978; 119:1408.

Block, G., Dresser, C. and Hartman, A., 'Nutrient sources in the American diet', *American Journal of Epidemiology*, 1985; 122:17–40.

Garrison, R.H. and Somer, E., *The Nutritional Desk Reference*, Keats Publishing Inc., Connecticut, 1990; xiii–xiv.

Hubert, H., Feinleib, M. and McNamara, P., 'Obesity as an

independent risk factor for cardiovascular disease – a 26 year follow up of participants in the Framingham Heart Study', *Circulation*, 1983; 67:968–77.

Salmon, J., *Dietary Reference Values*, Department of Health, London, 1991.

Trimmer, E.J., *The Complete Book of Slimming and Diets*, Piatkus, London, 1987.

Werback, M.R., *Nutriotional Influences on Illness*, Third Line Press Inc., New Canaan, Connecticut, 1988.

PART ONE

Garlic

Auer, W. *et al*, 'Hypertension and hyperlipidaemia: garlic helps in mild cases', *British Journal of Clinical Practice*, 1990; (s) 44, 8:3–7.

Greenwood, T.W. (ed.), 'Garlic Therapy', *British Journal of Clinical Practice*, 1990 (S) 69; 44, 8:1–39.

Vorbug, G. *et al*, 'Therapy with garlic; results of a placebo controlled double blind study', *British Journal of Clinical Practice*, 1990 (S) 44, 8:7–11.

Herbalist Products

Jarvis, D.C., *Folk Medicine*, W.H. Allen, London, 1960.

Nice, J., Herbal Remedies, Piatkus, London, 1990.

Magnesium

Durlach, J., *Magnesium in Clinical Practice*, John Libbey & Co., London, 1988.

Seelig, M., *Magnesium Deficiency in the Pathogenesis of Disease*, Plenum Medical, New York, 1980.

Trimmer, E.J., *The Magic of Magnesium*, Thorsons Publishing Group, Wellingborough, 1987.

Pollen, Propolis, Royal Jelly and the Bioflavonoids

Thorsons Editorial Board, *The Healing Power of Pollen*, Thorsons Publishing Group, Wellingborough, 1987.

Trimmer, E.J., 'The Bioflavonoids' (Vitamin P), in Barker, B.M. and Bender, B.A. (eds), *Vitamins in Medicine*, Heinemann, London, 1982; Vol. 2, 199–211.

Silicon

Edwardson, J.A. *et al*, 'Effect of silicon on absorption of aluminium', *Lancet*, 1993; 342: 211–12:

The Vitamins

Barker, B.M. and Bender, B.A. (eds), *Vitamins in Medicine*, Heinemann, London, 1982.

Mervyn, L., *The Dictionary of Vitamins*, Thorsons Publishing Group, Wellingborough, 1984.

Sinclair, H.M. and Hollingsworth, D.F., *Hutchinson's Food and the Principles of Nutrition*, Edward Arnold, London, 1969.

Truswell, A.S., 'Vitamins', *British Medical Journal,* 1985; 22:1103–6.

Zinc

Bryce-Smith, D. and Hodgkinson, L., *The Zinc Solution*, Century Arrow, London, 1986.

PART TWO

Acne

Bryce-Smith, D. and Hodgkinson, L., *The Zinc Solution*, Century Arrow, London, 1986.

Michaelsson, G. *et al*, 'A double blind study of zinc and oxytetracycline in acne vulgaris', *British Journal of Dermatology*, 1977; 97:561.

Michaelsson, G. *et al*, 'Erythrocyte glutathione activity in acne', *Acta Dermatology and Veneriology*, Stockholm, 1984; 64 (1):9 – 14.

Pohit, J. *et al*, 'Zinc status in acne vulgaris patients', *Journal of Applied Nutrition*, 1985; 37(1):18 – 25.

Alzheimer's Disease

Edwardson, J.A. *et al*, 'Effect of Silicon on absorption of aluminium', *Lancet*, 1993; 342:211 – 12.

Anaemia

Bernat, I., 'Iron deficiency' in *Iron Metabolism*, Plenum Press, New York, 1983.

Kemm, J.R. and Ancil, R.J., *Vitamin Deficiency in the Elderly*, Blackwell Scientific Publications, Oxford, 1985.

Kumar, J. and Clark, M.L., *Clinical Medicine,* Baillière Tindall, London, 1987.

Artery Problems

Kinsella, J. *et al*, 'Dietary Omega 3 polyunsaturated fatty acids and amelioration of cardiovascular disease – possible mechanisms', *American Journal of Clinical Nutrition*, 1990; 52:1 – 28.

Leaf, A. *et al,* 'Cardiovascular effects of Omega 3 fatty acids,', *New England Journal of Medicine,* 1988; 318:9, 349 – 57.

Monsink, R.P. *et al*, 'Effect of monounsaturated fats', *Lancet*, 1987; I: 122 – 5.

Salonen, J.T. *et al*, 'Association between cardiovascular death and myocardial infarction and serum selenium', *Lancet*, 1982; 2:175 – 9.

Saynor, R. *et al*, 'The long-term effects of dietary supplementation with fish oil concentrate', *Atherosclerosis*, 1984; 50:3 – 10.

Saynor, R. and Ryan, F., *The Eskimo Diet*, Ebury Press, London, 1990.

Truswell, A.S., 'Reducing the risk of coronary heart disease', *British Medical Journal*, 1985; 291: July 6.

Virtamo, J. *et al*, 'Serum selenium and risk of coronary heart disease and stroke', *American Journal of Epidemiology*, 1985; 122:276–82.

Arthritis and Rheumatism

Diplock, A.T., 'The role of antioxidants in clinical practice', *British Journal of Clinical Practice*, 1990; 44:257–9.

Kremer, J.H. *et al*, 'The effect of manipulation of dietary fatty acid on clinical manifestations of rheumatoid arthritis', *Lancet*, 1985; I:184–7.

Lewis, A., *Selenium*, Thorsons Publishing Group, Wellingborough, 1983.

Passwater, R.A., *Selenium as Food and Medicine*, Keats Publishing Inc., Connecticut, 1980.

Rudin, D., *The Omega 3 Phenomenon*, Sidgwick & Jackson, London, 1987.

Birth Defects (Spina Bifida)

MCR Research Group, 'Prevention of neural tube defects', *Lancet*, 1991; 338:131–7.

Cancer

Butterworth, C.E. *et al*, 'Improvement in cervical dysplasia associated with folic acid therapy in users of oral contraceptives', *American Journal of Clinical Nutrition*, 1982; 35:73–82.

Cahill, R.J. *et al*, 'Cell kinetic effects of Vitamin E and selenium supplementation in patients with adenomatous polyps', *European Journal of Cancer Prevention*, 1991; (S) 1:27–8.

Cahill, R.J. *et al*, 'Effects of selenium and Vitamin E supplementation on the colonic cell proliferation in patients with adenomatous polyps', *GUT*, 1991; 32(10):1235.

Graham, S. *et al*, 'Dietary factors in cancer of larynx', *American Journal of Epidemiology*, 1981; 113:675–80.

Menkes, U.S., 'Serum beta-carotene Vitamins A and E and selenium and the risk of lung cancer', *New England Journal of Medicine*, 1986; 313:1250.

Orr, J.W. *et al*, 'Plasma beta-carotene significantly lower in cancer patients', *American Journal of Obstetrics and Gynaecology*, 1985; 151:632–5.

Skekelle, R.B. *et al*, 'Dietary Vitamin A and cancer', *Lancet*, 1981; II:1185–90.

Willett, W.C. *et al*, 'Diet and cancer', *New England Journal of Medicine*, 1984; II:697–703.

Carpal Tunnel Syndrome

Scheyer, R.D., 'Pyridoxine in patients with carpal tunnel syndrome', Lancet, 1985; 2:42.

Cataract

Hankinson, S.E. *et al*, 'Nutrient intake and cataract extraction in women, a prospective study', *British Medical Journal*, 1992; 305:335–9.

Trevor-Roper, P.D., *Ophthalmology*, The Pocket Consultant series, Blackwell Scientific Publications, Oxford, 1985.

Colds

Eby, G.E. *et al*, 'Reduction in the duration of common colds by zinc gluconate lozenges in a double blind study', *Antimicrobiological Agents and Chemotherapy*, 1984; 25 (I): 20–24.

Peretz, A. *et al*, 'Lymphocyte response is enhanced by

supplementation of elderly subjects with selenium-enriched yeast', *American Journal of Clinical Nutrition*, 1991; 53: 1323 – 8.

Constipation

Handler, S., 'Dietary fibre: can it prevent certain colonic diseases?', *Postgraduate Medicine*, 1973; 301 – 7.

Crohn's Disease and Ulcerative Colitis

Grimes, D.S., 'Refined carbohydrate, smooth muscle spasm and disease of the colon', *Lancet*, 1976; I:395 – 7.
Heaton, K.W. *et al*, 'Treatment of Crohn's disease', *British Medical Journal*, 1979; 2:764 – 6.

O'Morain, C. *et al*, 'Elemental diet in acute Crohn's disease', *Archives of Diseases of Childhood*, 1983; 53:44 (observational study).

Diabetes

Philipson, H., 'Dietary fibre in the diabetic diet', *Acta Medicina Scandinavia*, 1983 (S); 671:91 – 3.

Trowell, H.C., 'Dietary fibre hypothesis of the aetiology of diabetes mellitus', *Diabetes*, 1975; 24(8):762 – 5.

Vogelsang, A., 'Vitamin E may reduce insulin requirement', *Annals of the New York Academy of Science*, 1949; 52:406.

Dysmenorrhoea

Abraham, C.E., 'Primary dysmenorrhoea', *Clinics in Obstetrics and Gynaecology*, 1978; 21 (i):139 – 45.

Butler, E.B. *et al*, 'Vitamin B in the treatment of primary dysmenorrhoea', *Lancet*, 1955; I:844 – 7.

Hudgins, A.P., 'Vitamins A, C and niacin for dysmenorrhoea', *Western Journal of Surgery and Gynaecology*, 1954; 62:610 – 11.

Eczema

Graham, J., *Evening Primrose Oil*, Thorsons Publishing Group, Wellingborough, 1989.

Manku, M.S. *et al*, 'Reduced levels of prostaglandin precursors in the blood of atopic patients', *Prostaglandins, Leukotrienes and Medicine*, 1982; 9(6):615–28.

Wright, S. *et al*, 'Oral evening primrose oil improves atopic eczema', *Lancet*, 1982; II: 1120–22.

Fibrocystic Breast Disease

Boyle, L.A. *et al*, 'Caffeine consumption and fibrocystic breast disease – a case control epidemiological study', *Journal Canadian Nutriotional Institute* 1984; 77(3):1015–199.

Pye, J.K. *et al*, 'Clinical experience of drug treatments for mastalgia', *Lancet*, 1985; 2:373–7.

Gall Bladder Problems

Bell, G.D. *et al*, 'Gallstone dissolution in man using an essential oil preparation', *British Medical Journal*, 1979; I:24.

McDougall, R.M. *et al*, 'The effect of added bran on the saturation of bile in people without gallstones', *American Journal of Surgery*, 1978; 135:321.

Pixley, F. *et al*, 'Effect of vegetarianism on development of gallstones', *British Medical Journal*, 1985; 291:11–12.

Scragg, R.K.R. *et al*, 'Refined sugar intake a risk factor independent of obesity', *British Medical Journal*, 1984; 288:1113.

Thornton, J.R. *et al*, 'Diet and gallstones', *GUT*, 1983; 24:2–6.

Herpes

Finnerty, E.F., 'Topical zinc in the treatment of herpes simplex', *Cutis*, 1986; 37:(2)130.

Fitzherbert, J., letter to editor, *Medical Journal of Australia*, 1979; 1:399.

Oates, J.K., *Herpes, The Facts,* Penguin Books, London, 1983.

Skinner, G.R.B., 'Lithium ointment for genital herpes', *Lancet*, 1983; 2:288.

Terezhalmy, G.T., 'Water-soluble bioflavonoid complex in the treatment of recurrent herpes labialis', *Oral Surgery, Oral Medicine, Oral Pathology*, 1978; 45:56–62.

Hyperkinesis

Brenner, A., 'Effects of mega doses of selected B complex vitamins on children with hyperkinesis', *Journal of Learning Disabilities*, 1982; 15:258.

Colquhoun, I. *et al*, 'A lack of EFAs as a possible cause of hyperactivity in children', *Medical Hypotheses*, 1981; 7: 673–9.

Eggar, J. *et al*, 'Controlled trial of oligo antigenic treatment in the hyperkinetic child', *Lancet*, 1985; I:540–45.

Heffer, A., 'Vitamin B 3 dependent child', *Schizophrenia*, 1971; 3:107–13.

Hodgkinson, L., 'Overactive ingredients in boys and girls', *The Times*, 8 August 1991.

Kaplan, H.K. *et al*, 'Behavioural effects of dietary sucrose in disturbed children', *American Journal of Psychiatry*, 1986; 143 (7):944–5.

Hypertension

Burr, H.L. *et al*, 'Dietary fibre blood pressure and blood cholesterol', *Nutritional Reviews*, 1985; 5:465–72.

Khaw, K.T. *et al*, 'Randomised double blind crossover trial of potassium on blood pressure in normal subjects', *Lancet*, 1982; 2:1127–9.

Le Fanu, J., *Eat Your Heart Out*, Macmillan Papermac, London, 1987.

Norris, P.G. *et al*, 'Effect of dietary supplementation with fish oil on systolic blood pressure in mild essential hypertension', *British Medical Journal*, 1986; 243:104.

Immunodepression

Alexander, M. *et al*, letter to the editor, 'Oral beta-carotene can increase number of T4 cells in human blood', *Immunology* (letters), 1985; 9:221–4.

Chandra, R.K., 'Trace element regulation of immunity and infection', *Journal of the American College of Nutrition*, 1985; 4 (i):5–16.

Diplock, A.T., letter to the editor, *Journal of Nutritional Medicine*, 1991; 2:209–11.

Levy, J.E., 'Nutrition and the immune system', *Basic and Clinical Immunology*, 1982; 297–305.

Irritable Bowel Syndrome

Kruis, W. *et al*, 'Comparison of wheatbran, mebeverine and placebo in patients with IBS', *Digestion*, 1956; 34:196.

Rees, W.R.W. *et al*, 'Treating IBS with peppermint oil', *British Medical Journal*, 1979; 2:835–836.

Soltoft, J., *et al*, 'A double blind trial of the effects of wheat bran on symptoms of IBS', *Lancet*, 1976; I: 270–72.

Kidney Stones

Trimmer, E.J., *The Magic of Magnesium*, Thorsons Publishing Group, Wellingborough, 1987.

Menopausal Problems

Finken, R.S., 'The effect of Vitamin E in the menopause', *Journal of Clinical Endocrinology and Metabolism*, 1949; 9:89–94.

Werbach, M.R., *Nutritional Influences on Illness*, Third Line Press, Keats Publishing Inc., Connecticut, 1987.

Menorrhagia

Taymor, M.L. *et al*, 'The aetiological role of chronic iron deficiency in production of menorrhagia', *Journal of the American Medical Association*, 1964; 187:323–7.

Multiple Sclerosis

Dworkin, R.H., 'Linoleic acid and multiple sclerosis', *Lancet*, 1981; I:1153–4.

Field, E.J. *et al*, 'Multiple sclerosis: effect of gamma-linoleic and the need for extended clinical trials on unsaturated fatty acids', *European Neurology*, 1983; 22:78.

Swank, R.L., 'Multiple sclerosis, 20 years on a low-fat diet', *Archives of Neurology*, 1970; 23:460–74.

Periodontal Disease

Bliznakov, E.G., *The Miracle Nutrient Coenzyme Q10*, Bantam Books, New York, 1987.

Folkers, K. *et al*, review article, *Biomedical and Clinical Aspects of Coenzyme Q*', Amsterdam Elsevier/North Holland, Biomedical Press, 1977; 1:294–311.

Hanson, I.L. *et al*, 'Gingival and leucocytic deficiencies of Coenzyme Q10 in patients with periodontal disease', *Reviews and Communications in Chemical Pathology and Pharmacology*, 1976; 14:729.

Pre-Menstrual Syndrome

Abraham, G.E., 'Nutritional factors in the aetiology of the premenstrual syndrome', *Journal of Reproductive Medicine*, 1983; 28 (7):446–64.

Brush, M.G. *et al*, 'Pyridoxine and PMS', *Lancet*, 1985; I: 1339.

Harding Branch, C.H., *Aspects of Anxiety*, Lippincott, Philadelphia, 1965.

Williams, M.J. *et al*, 'Controlled trial of pyridoxine in PMS', *Journal of Internal Medicine Review*, 1985; 13:174–9.

Prostatitis and Prostate Problems

Buck, A.C. *et al*, 'Treatment of outflow tract obstruction due to benign prostatic hyperplasia with the pollen extract Cernilton – a double blind placebo controlled study', *British Journal of Urology*, 1990; 66:398–404.

Rugendorff, E.W. *et al*, Results of treatment with pollen extract (Cernilton) in chronic prostatitis', *British Journal of Urology*, 1993; 71:433–8.

Rickets

Garrison, R.H. Somer, E., *The Nutritional Desk Reference*, Keats Publishing, New Canaan, Connecticut, 1990.

Hughes, J.G., *Synopsis of Pediatrics*, C V Mosby Co, St. Louis, 1984.

Tension and Stress

Davies. S., Stewart, A. *Nutritional Medicine*, Pan Books, London, 1987; London

Trimmer, E.J., *Good Housekeeping Guide to Medicines*, Ebury Press, London, 1983.

Tiredness and Fatigue

Van der Beek, E.J., *'Vitamins and edndurance training'*, Sports Medicine, 1985; 2(3):175–197.

Charaskin E. *'Daily Vitamin C consumption and fatigability'*, Journal American Geriatric Soc., 1976; 24(3); 1936–7.

Blizmakov, E.G., Hunt, G.L. *The Miracle Nutrient Coenzyme Q10*, Bantam, New York, 1989.

Varicose Veins, Ulcers and Haemorrhoids

Greaves, M.W. *et al 'Effects of Long continued ingestion of zinc sulphate in patients with various leg ulceration'*, Lancet, 1970; 30: 889–891.

Bryce-Smith, D., Hodgkinson, L., *The Zinc Solution* Century Arrow, London, 1986.

Stanway, A., *Taking the Rough with the Smooth*, Souvenir Press, London, 1976.

INDEX

Page numbers in **bold** *type indicate main references*